Clinical Nutrition

Editors

DOTTIE LAFLAMME
DEBRA L. ZORAN

VETERINARY CLINICS OF NORTH AMERICA: SMALL ANIMAL PRACTICE

www.vetsmall.theclinics.com

July 2014 • Volume 44 • Number 4

ELSEVIER

1600 John F. Kennedy Boulevard • Suite 1800 • Philadelphia, Pennsylvania, 19103-2899

http://www.vetsmall.theclinics.com

VETERINARY CLINICS OF NORTH AMERICA: SMALL ANIMAL PRACTICE Volume 44, Number 4

July 2014 ISSN 0195-5616, ISBN-13: 978-0-323-31176-2

Editor: Patrick Manley

Developmental Editor: Susan Showalter

Veterinary Clinics of North America: Small Animal Practice (ISSN 0195-5616) is published bimonthly by Elsevier Inc., 360 Park Avenue South, New York, NY 10010-1710. Months of issue are January, March, May, July, September, and November. Business and Editorial Offices: 1600 John F. Kennedy Blvd., Ste. 1800, Philadelphia, PA 19103-2899. Customer Service Office: 3251 Riverport Lane, Maryland Heights, MO 63043. Periodicals postage paid at New York, NY and additional mailing offices. Subscription prices are $310.00 per year (domestic individuals), $500.00 per year (domestic institutions), $150.00 per year (domestic students/residents), $410.00 per year (Canadian individuals), $621.00 per year (Canadian institutions), $455.00 per year (international individuals), $621.00 per year (international institutions), and $220.00 per year (international and Canadian students/residents). To receive student/resident rate, orders must be accompanied by name of affiliated institution, date of term, and the *signature* of program/residency coordinator on institution letterhead. Orders will be billed at individual rate until proof of status is received. Foreign air speed delivery is included in all *Clinics* subscription prices. All prices are subject to change without notice. **POSTMASTER:** Send address changes to *Veterinary Clinics of North America: Small Animal Practice*, Elsevier Health Sciences Division, Subscription Customer Service, 3251 Riverport Lane, Maryland Heights, MO 63043. Customer Service (orders, claims, online, change of address): Elsevier Periodicals Customer Service, Elsevier Health Sciences Division Subscription Customer Service 3251 Riverport Lane Maryland Heights, MO 63043. Tel: 1-800-654-2452 (U.S. and Canada); 314-447-8871 (outside U.S. and Canada). Fax: 314-447-8029. E-mail: journalscustomerservice-usa@elsevier.com (for print support); journalsonlinesupport-usa@elsevier.com (for online support).

Reprints. For copies of 100 or more of articles in this publication, please contact the Commercial Reprints Department, Elsevier Inc., 360 Park Avenue South, New York, NY 10010-1710. Tel.: 212-633-3874; Fax: 212-633-3820; E-mail: reprints@elsevier.com.

Veterinary Clinics of North America: Small Animal Practice is also published in Japanese by Inter Zoo Publishing Co., Ltd., Aoyama Crystal-Bldg 5F, 3-5-12 Kitaaoyama, Minato-ku, Tokyo 107-0061, Japan.

Veterinary Clinics of North America: Small Animal Practice is covered in *Current Contents/Agriculture, Biology and Environmental Sciences, Science Citation Index, ASCA, MEDLINE/PubMed (Index Medicus), Excerpta Medica,* and *BIOSIS.*

Contributors

EDITORS

DOTTIE LAFLAMME, DVM, PhD
Diplomate, American College of Veterinary Nutrition; Nestlé Purina Research, St Louis, Missouri

DEBRA L. ZORAN, DVM, PhD, DACVIM
Department of Small Animal Clinical Sciences, College of Veterinary Medicine & Biomedical Sciences, Texas A&M University, College Station, Texas

AUTHORS

STEPHEN BINDER, PhD
Product Technology Center, Nestlé Purina PetCare Company, St Louis, Missouri

MARJORIE L. CHANDLER, DVM, MS, MRCVS
Private Consultant, Lasswade, Midlothian; Honorary Senior Lecturer, The Royal (Dick) School of Veterinary Studies, University of Edinburgh, Roslin, Scotland

LAURA EIRMANN, DVM
Diplomate, American College of Veterinary Nutrition; Oradell Animal Hospital, Paramus; Nestlé Purina PetCare Company, Ringwood, New Jersey; Nestlé Purina PetCare Company, St Louis, Missouri

AMY FARCAS, DVM, MS
Diplomate, American College of Veterinary Nutrition; Lecturer in Clinical Nutrition, Department of Clinical Studies, School of Veterinary Medicine, University of Pennsylvania, Philadelphia, Pennsylvania

ANDREA J. FASCETTI, VMD, PhD
Diplomate, American College of Veterinary Internal Medicine (Small Animal); Diplomate, American College of Veterinary Nutrition; Professor, Department of Molecular Biosciences, University of California Davis, Davis, California

DANIÈLLE GUNN-MOORE, BVM&S, PhD, MRCVS, RCVS Specialist in Feline Medicine
Professor of Feline Medicine, Royal (Dick) School of Veterinary Studies and The Roslin Institute, The University of Edinburgh, Roslin, Scotland

OSCAR IZQUIERDO, PhD
Product Technology Center, Nestlé Purina PetCare Company, St Louis, Missouri

DOTTIE LAFLAMME, DVM, PhD
Diplomate, American College of Veterinary Nutrition; Nestlé Purina Research, St Louis, Missouri

JENNIFER A. LARSEN, DVM, PhD
Diplomate, American College of Veterinary Nutrition; Assistant Professor of Clinical Nutrition, VM: Molecular Biosciences, School of Veterinary Medicine, University of California, Davis, Davis, California

DEBORAH LINDER, DVM
Diplomate, American College of Veterinary Nutrition; Department of Clinical Sciences, Cummings School of Veterinary Medicine at Tufts University, North Grafton, Massachusetts

MEGAN MUELLER, PhD
Center for Animals and Public Policy, Cummings School of Veterinary Medicine at Tufts University, North Grafton, Massachusetts

JACQUELINE M. PARR, DVM, MSc
Post-Doctoral Fellow in Clinical Nutrition, Clinical Nutrition Service, Department of Clinical Studies, Ontario Veterinary College, University of Guelph; Owner of On Parr Nutrition, Inc, Guelph, Ontario, Canada

MARK E. PETERSON, DVM
Diplomate, American College of Veterinary Internal Medicine; Adjunct Professor of Medicine, Department of Clinical Sciences, New York State College of Veterinary Medicine, Cornell University, Ithaca; Animal Endocrine Clinic, New York, New York

REBECCA L. REMILLARD, PhD, DVM
Diplomate, American College of Veterinary Nutrition; Nutrition Service, Clinical Veterinarian, Small and Large Animal Nutrition, Molecular Biomedical Science Department, College of Veterinary Medicine, North Carolina State University, Raleigh; Owner of Veterinary Nutritional Consultations, Inc, Hollister, North Carolina; Consultant Rayne Clinical Nutrition LLC, Kansas City, Missouri

JUSTIN SHMALBERG, DVM
Diplomate, American College of Veterinary Nutrition; Department of Clinical Sciences, University of Florida, Gainesville, Florida

GREGG TAKASHIMA, DVM
Medical Director, The Parkway Veterinary Hospital; President, GKT Enterprises, PC, Lake Oswego, Oregon

CECILIA VILLAVERDE, BVSc, PhD
Diplomate, American College of Veterinary Nutrition; Diplomate, European College of Veterinary and Comparative Nutrition; Adjunct Professor, Departament de Ciència Animal i dels Aliments (Animal and Food Science Department), Universitat Autònoma de Barcelona, Bellaterra, Spain

JOSEPH WAKSHLAG, DVM, PhD
Diplomate, American College of Veterinary Nutrition; Diplomate, American College of Veterinary Sports Medicine and Rehabilitation; Department of Clinical Sciences, College of Veterinary Medicine, Cornell University, Ithaca, New York

Contents

Although veterinary practitioners know that nutrition can make a difference in the health and recovery from disease or illness in dogs and cats, they may feel poorly equipped to provide unbiased information on nutrition. This article provides information about evaluating and recommending diets and interpreting a pet food label to allow for comparisons among pet foods and discussion about how to do a nutritional assessment. It provides an example of how nutritional assessment and recommendation were successfully introduced into a busy private practice. Finally, some of the myths and misperceptions about nutrition are discussed with information provided from evidence-based research.

The goal of this article was to provide veterinary practitioners with an overview of the types of alternative dietary options available to pet owners and a practical method by which to evaluate the nutritional adequacy of these various options. Our approach to categorizing the alternative dietary options is based on the nutritional adequacy of these dietary options, because patients will be at risk for nutrition-related diseases if fed a nutritionally incomplete or improperly balanced diet long term.

Information and misinformation about pet nutrition and pet foods, including ingredients used in pet foods, is widely available through various sources. Often, this "information" raises questions or concerns among pet owners. Many pet owners will turn to their veterinarian for answers to these questions. One of the challenges that veterinarians have is keeping up with the volume of misinformation about pet foods and sorting out fact from fiction. The goal of this article is to provide facts regarding some common myths about ingredients used in commercial pet foods so as to better prepare veterinarians to address their client's questions.

Dietary macronutrients include protein, fat, and carbohydrates. Current nutritional recommendations establish minimums but not maximums for protein and fat but not for carbohydrates; thus, commercial feline

addressed. However, nutritional support can play an integral role in the successful management of feline endocrine diseases. Furthermore, because most cats with endocrine disease are senior or geriatric, they may also have concurrent health conditions that warrant dietary intervention. This article discusses recommendations for nutritional support of the 2 most common endocrine problems of cats seen in clinical practice: hyperthyroidism and diabetes mellitus.

 Video of successful weight management strategy in an 8-year-old dog accompanies this article

Excess weight has been associated with many clinical and subclinical conditions that put a pet's health at risk. Successful weight management programs extend beyond standard nutritional management and incorporate an understanding of human-animal interaction. Understanding the processes and dynamics of human-animal relationships can be a useful tool for practitioners in developing successful treatment plans for their clients. Obesity is a nutritional disorder requiring lifelong management; however, when veterinarians go beyond standard treatment to include an understanding of human-animal interaction, it is also one of the few conditions in veterinary medicine that is completely preventable and curable.

VETERINARY CLINICS OF NORTH AMERICA: SMALL ANIMAL PRACTICE

RELATED INTEREST

Veterinary Clinics of North America: Exotic Animal Practice
September 2014, Volume 17, Number 3
Nutrition
Jörg Mayer, *Editor*

THE CLINICS ARE NOW AVAILABLE ONLINE!
Access your subscription at:
www.theclinics.com

Preface

Clinical Nutrition

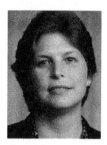 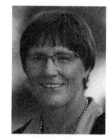

Dottie Laflamme, DVM, PhD, DACVN   Debra L. Zoran, DVM, PhD, DACVIM
Editors

Good nutrition plays an important role in preventive health care, as well as in the management of various medical conditions. But delivering good nutrition means different things to different people. Veterinarians remain the number one source of information about nutrition for the majority of pet owners, although other sources, such as the internet, are gaining in popularity and influence. As such, it is imperative that veterinarians develop a good working knowledge about nutrition and apply this knowledge to their daily practice. The World Small Animal Veterinary Association and the American Animal Hospital Association have partnered with various groups and industry partners to not only encourage veterinarians to incorporate nutritional assessments into every patient evaluation but also provide tools to make it easier to do so. This issue of *Veterinary Clinics of North America: Small Animal Practice* does not repeat what is available elsewhere, but provides valuable resources, tools, and information to supplement what is otherwise available.

The topics covered in this issue reflect the fact that the majority of pet dogs and cats seen by veterinarians are healthy or generally healthy, yet may have different nutritional needs. Some pet owners prefer to feed commercial pet foods, while others prefer other options. Separate articles here provide insights that will help veterinarians feel more confident when evaluating home-prepared foods or evaluating commercial pet foods.

In recent years, there has been considerable debate over the unique dietary needs of cats. Particularly of interest is the relative value of proteins and carbohydrates in feline diets. Likewise, working and service dogs, and aging dogs and cats, all can have special dietary needs. Separate articles herein address each of these issues.

This issue concludes with articles addressing common diet-sensitive problems: endocrine diseases in cats, and obesity in cats and dogs. Obesity is considered the most common form of malnutrition in developed countries, and controlling obesity can be challenging. This article provides information that goes beyond simple dietary issues and addresses some of the communications and environmental needs required to effectively manage pet obesity.

Vet Clin Small Anim 44 (2014) ix–x
http://dx.doi.org/10.1016/j.cvsm.2014.05.001
0195-5616/14/$ – see front matter © 2014 Elsevier Inc. All rights reserved.

We thank the contributing authors for providing their time, expertise, and valuable viewpoints. We believe that every small animal veterinarian will find this issue of *Veterinary Clinics of North America: Small Animal Practice* to be very useful. We encourage you to use these resources to build your confidence and increase your practice of performing nutritional assessments and providing sound nutritional advice for your patients.

Dottie Laflamme, DVM, PhD, DACVN
Nestlé Purina Research
Checkerboard Square
St. Louis, MO 63164, USA

Debra L. Zoran, DVM, PhD, DACVIM
Department of Small Animal Clinical Sciences
College of Veterinary Medicine & Biomedical Sciences
Texas A&M University
College Station, TX 77843-4474, USA

E-mail addresses:
Dorothy.laflamme@rd.nestle.com (D. Laflamme)
DZORAN@cvm.tamu.edu (D.L. Zoran)

Nutritional Concepts for the Veterinary Practitioner

Marjorie L. Chandler, DVM, MS, MRCVS[a,b,*], Gregg Takashima, DVM[c]

KEYWORDS

- Pet food labels • Nutritional assessment • Body condition score • Muscle condition
- Nutritional myths

KEY POINTS

- Diet may help treat, or decrease the risk of, disease, or cause it if there are problems with the food or feeding management.
- To evaluate pet foods, practitioners should be aware of what nutrient requirements have been used to formulate the diet and if it has been tested by computer, chemical analysis, and/or feeding trials.
- The nutrient analysis on pet foods may be used to compare foods if they are compared on an energy or dry-matter basis.
- When recommending a diet to the owner, the practitioner should ensure that it is complete and balanced, have adequate digestibility, and is safe. High-quality diets may have ingredients with added health benefits.
- A screening nutritional assessment should be performed for every pet at every veterinary visit.

INTRODUCTION

Nutrition for the general veterinary practitioner is often not fully incorporated into veterinary or veterinary nursing school curriculums or recognized by the profession. Every practitioner and nurse have seen how nutrition can make a difference for their patients, but they often lack the tools needed to make an informed recommendation because there is often a confusing mix of, or insufficient, information available.

To complicate things further, veterinarians often sell certain brands of diets and the profits may contribute significantly to the practice income. Thus, recommendations for that particular veterinary practice–carried diet, no matter how appropriate, may be met with suspicion from the public, who are also confronted with confusing and sometimes misleading nutritional information.

[a] Private Consultant, 11 Mavisbank Place, Lasswade, Midlothian EH18 1DQ, Scotland; [b] The Royal (Dick) School of Veterinary Studies, University of Edinburgh, Roslin, Scotland; [c] The Parkway Veterinary Hospital, GKT Enterprises, PC, 3 Southwest Monroe Parkway, Suite Y, Lake Oswego, OR 97035, USA
* Corresponding author. Private Consultant, 11 Mavisbank Place, Lasswade, Midlothian EH18 1DQ, Scotland.
E-mail address: m.chandler@ed.ac.uk

Vet Clin Small Anim 44 (2014) 645–666
http://dx.doi.org/10.1016/j.cvsm.2014.03.009
0195-5616/14/$ – see front matter © 2014 Elsevier Inc. All rights reserved.

Compounding this is the fragmentation of the profession surrounding nutritional concepts: for example, some favoring raw-food or homemade diets versus commercially prepared foods, and some favoring or discounting foods based on retail location or type, such as grocery stores or veterinary practices.

DISEASES AND NUTRITION

Many diseases are influenced by nutrition. These diseases can include nutrient-sensitive diseases, diet-induced diseases, and food or feeding management problems. A nutrient-sensitive disease is one in which the pet's disorder may benefit from a special diet as part of the therapy, for example, chronic kidney disease, some hepatopathies, feline diabetes, and many types of gastrointestinal disease (**Box 1**).[1] A diet-induced disease is a problem that is caused by the diet. This problem can be caused by formulation errors resulting in deficiencies or excesses of nutrients, a problem very common in homemade diets that have not been balanced (**Fig. 1**),[2] and also occurs in commercial diets. Processing errors may also occur, resulting in destruction of nutrients or inappropriate addition of excessive or deficient amounts of nutrients. These processing errors also include the presence of toxins and bacterial contamination, which have been especially reported in raw diets (commercial or homemade) but also in commercial cooked pet foods.[3]

One of the best known cases of diet contamination was in 2007, when unscrupulous suppliers in China added the contaminants melamine and cyanuric acid to increase the apparent protein levels in food-grade wheat gluten and rice protein concentrate. The adulterated ingredients ended up in foods and treats made by 12 different pet food manufacturers, according to court documents. Tens of thousands of animals ate the contaminated foods, and many became sick, some fatally. Although neither melamine nor cyanuric acid is toxic individually, the combination of melamine and cyanuric acid forms crystals in the kidneys, potentially leading to kidney failure. The pet food industry reacted quickly by calling for the biggest pet food recall in history and

---

Box 1
Common disorders that may be nutrient sensitive

Dental disease

Diabetes mellitus

Hyperlipidemia

Obesity

Gastrointestinal disorders

Pancreatitis

Liver disorders

Heart disease

Kidney disease

Dermatopathies

Urolithiasis

Osteoarthritis

Cognitive disorders

Feline thyroid disease

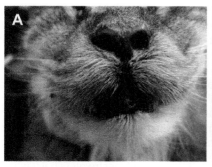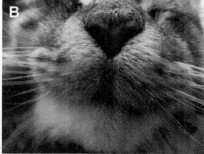

Fig. 1. A 2-year-old Maine Coon cat on an unbalanced homemade diet (*A*) and after the diet had been improved (*B*). (*Courtesy of* Dr Elise Robertson, Brighton, England.)

steps were been taken by both the industry and the US Food and Drug Administration (FDA) to reduce the risks for similar problems in the future.[4,5]

After processing, the food may be stored incorrectly, potentially resulting in stale, moldy, or infested foods or a decrease in nutrients (see Nutritional Assessment section for more on feeding management).

EVALUATION OF PET FOODS

Veterinarians and pet owners are often unsure how to evaluate a pet food, or to determine if the added cost of a food is worthwhile. Pet foods do differ in quality, and the most basic requirement is that the diet is complete and balanced in required nutrients. A complete food provides adequate amounts of all required nutrients. The term balanced is usually used in conjunction with complete and means the food has all the nutrients present in the proper proportions.[6]

There are several standards for requirements for the nutrients in pet food, including the Association of American Feed Control Officials (AAFCO),[7] the National Research Council (NRC),[8] and the European Pet Food Federation.[9] Compliance with these standards is generally voluntary; however, within the United States, AAFCO's guidelines are the basis for most state's pet food regulations. Foods sold in those states must comply with the adopted regulations regarding nutritional standards and labeling guidelines. Outside of states that comply with AAFCO regulations, most legislation concerns labeling and does not guarantee the completeness or safety of the food.

Pet foods can be tested for adequacy in *at least* 1 of 3 ways: (1) computerized analysis or calculation, (2) chemical analysis, and (3) feeding trials. Computer analysis is the most basic way to design a diet and is the starting point for developing a diet. Computer analysis or calculation determines (or estimates) the concentrations of required nutrients in a diet. Balancing a diet by computer or calculation will usually pick up large errors in formulation, but assumes, not always accurately, that the food products used in the diet have the same nutrients as the ones listed in the computer data base or in standard nutrient tables.[10]

Laboratory analysis of a finished food product gives a more accurate description of the nutrients than computer analysis, but is more costly. The laboratory analyses performed provide the proximate analysis of the food. This analysis includes percentages of moisture, protein, fat, ash (minerals), and fiber in the food. The soluble carbohydrates are estimated by subtraction of the other components from 100% and are termed nitrogen-free extract in the analysis. Individual minerals, vitamins, and amino acids may not be evaluated, although larger companies will often perform these analyses, and in US states that comply with AAFCO guidelines, these nutrients are either analyzed or calculated for those not evaluated in feeding trials. Interactions between nutrients, digestibility, and availability of nutrients, toxicities, and acceptability are not taken into account with either computer or laboratory analyses.

After a diet has been developed by computer analysis and checked by chemical analysis, feeding trials are recommended to test for digestibility, negative interference or interactions among nutrients, palatability, potential toxicities, or other problems that may show up when the diet is fed to animals. AAFCO has standards for feeding trials that many companies use. These trials evaluate parameters, such as body weight and measurements, evaluation of hair coat condition, and certain blood parameters. The age and life stage of the dog or cat used in the feeding trial must be consistent with the recommended use of the product. Feeding trials are considered to be a good evaluation of pet foods; however, the use of feeding trials does not guarantee the food provides adequate nutrition under all conditions or for longer than the duration of the trial. Many of the larger pet food companies do much more intensive, extensive, and longer feeding trials than the minimum set by AAFCO. This research provides vital nutrition information for the veterinary community as well as testing the diets.

Nutrient requirements may be stated in different ways. The NRC defines the minimum requirement for the animal as the minimal amount of a bioavailable nutrient that will support a defined physiologic state (eg, maintenance, growth, pregnancy, or lactation). An "adequate intake" is the concentration in the diet or amount required by the animal that is presumed to sustain a given life stage whereby no minimum requirement has been demonstrated. The "Recommended Allowance" is based on the minimum requirement, but is increased to take into account a bioavailability factor. For example, digestible energy may be determined by animal experiment or calculated with predictive equations. Originally, Atwater factors of 9 kcal/g and 4 kcal/g of protein and carbohydrate (estimated from nitrogen-free extract) were used to estimate metabolizable energy (ME). These ingredients work well in homemade diets such as meat or offal and use a digestibility of 98% for carbohydrates, 96% for fat, and 90% for protein, although the fat digestibility is likely overestimated for cats by a small amount.[8]

If the Atwater factors are used for processed diets for dogs or cats, they overestimate the ME; therefore, modified Atwater factors are used (ie, 8.5 kcal/g for fat and 3.5 kcal/g for protein and for carbohydrate). As the digestibility of commercial foods varies greatly, these factors may still not be accurate.[8,11,12]

For nutritionally balanced diets, the essential nutrients must be provided in proportion to the energy density of the diet. AAFCO guidelines, percentage basis, assume an ME of 4000 kcal/kg for cat foods and 3500 kcal/kg for dog foods, but this issue is eliminated in their guidelines listing nutrients per 1000 kcal ME. However, guidelines still are based on average energy intake. For dogs or cats with very low energy needs, the amount of food consumed will be reduced, and if a nutrient in the food is near the minimum requirement, the decreased intake could result in deficient intake of that nutrient. Therefore, it is important that pets be fed diets with energy densities suited to their energy requirements.

For many nutrients such as calcium and vitamins A and D, there is a safe upper limit (SUL), which is the maximum concentration or amount of a nutrient that has been tested and shown not to be associated with adverse effects.[8] In some cases, there are no data on which to establish an SUL because no detrimental effects have been noted at any level tested. Both the adequate or minimum amounts and the SUL of nutrients are potentially more crucial during growth.

HELPING OWNERS CHOOSE A DIET

Veterinarians may be asked by an owner, "What is the best food to feed my pet?" There is no one best pet food or pet food company for all pets. A nutritional assessment will provide a guideline for choice regarding age, breed, body condition, and the presence of disease. A minimum standard is a complete and balanced diet that has adequate digestibility, is sufficiently palatable to be eaten in appropriate quantities, and is free from toxins.[6] The choice of dry or canned forms of food is usually made because of owner preference and possibly cost, unless the animal has a requirement for higher fluid intake (eg, a cat with chronic kidney disease). Other considerations include the reputation of the company, if good feeding trials are performed, and if the company has strict quality control measures. The highest quality companies usually perform their own research and development and should be able to supply a nutrient-complete analysis for their pet foods. Many of the companies have performed research showing the benefits of added ingredients, and this may have a role in the choice of diet.[13]

PET FOOD LABELS

Pet food labels usually have 2 parts: the principal display panel and the information panel in the United States (US) or statutory statement in the European Union (EU). The principal display panel contains the brand name, product name, the statement of intent (only required in the US) (eg, "food for dogs"), the net weight, bursts or flags (eg, "NEW AND IMPROVED"), and probably a product picture or slogan. The information panel or statutory statement includes the ingredient statement, the typical (EU) or guaranteed (US) analysis, the product description, feeding guidelines, nutrient declaration, additives declaration, and manufacturer or distributor name and address. The ingredient statement is a list of the ingredients used in descending order of predominance by weight. In the United States, every ingredient must be listed separately either by its official name or by its common name.

In the European Union, the type of ingredient can be stated by an individual name or may be grouped under various categories as stipulated in the regulations. There are categories for meat and animal derivatives, derivatives of vegetable origin, milk and milk derivatives, and so forth.

The guaranteed analysis (US) lists the minimum amounts of crude protein, and crude fat, and the maximum amounts of moisture and crude fiber. The crude fat, protein, and fiber analyses refer to the specific analytical procedures that are used to estimate these nutrients. The procedures contain some inaccuracies, but are useful estimates and can be used for comparison of products. Note that these are maximums and minimums and not exact amounts. EU regulations dictate that the typical concentrations of protein, fat or oil, fiber, and ash be listed as percentages of the product. The percentage of moisture (water) must also be listed if it is greater than 14%.[10]

When evaluating a pet food, the moisture content should be taken into consideration. The nutrient levels on the label are on an "as-fed" basis, meaning that they include the moisture. Because pet foods may vary from about 8% to 80% moisture, this makes comparing them difficult, so pet foods are usually evaluated by nutritionists on a "dry-matter" or an "energy" basis. To calculate the amount of a food nutrient on a dry-matter basis, the percentage of moisture is subtracted from 100 to determine the amount of dry matter in the food. The as-fed percentage of a nutrient is then divided by the dry matter to determine the percentage of the nutrient on a dry-matter basis (**Box 2**).

Many nutritionists prefer to compare nutrients on an energy basis, because animals (should) eat an appropriate amount of calories; not taking this into account may cause incorrect assumptions about the animal's intake of a nutrient. For example, with

---

Box 2
Converting nutrients from as-fed to dry matter basis

To convert a nutrient from an as-fed to a dry-matter (DM) basis, first subtract the percentage of moisture from 100% to determine the percentage of DM, for example, for a dry food, this might be:

100% − 10% water = 90% DM

The percentage of the as-fed nutrient is then divided by the percentage of DM; for example, the above dry food diet with 20% protein on an as-fed basis:

20% as-fed protein ÷ 0.90 = 22.2% protein on a DMbasis.

Note 1: when calculating using percentages, the percentage is first divided by 100, so 90% becomes 0.90.

Note 2: the amount of a nutrient on a DM basis will always be larger than it is on the as-fed basis.

Note 3: remember to use the percentage of DM, not the percentage of moisture!

To convert from DM basis to as-fed basis, multiply by the percentage of DM, for example: 22.2% (DM) × 0.90 = 20.0% as fed

In contrast, a wet food containing 75% water (25% dry matter) and 10% protein on an as-fed basis would contain 10/0.25 or 40% protein on a DM basis.

---

a high-calorie, low-protein food, it may be possible for the animal to have an insufficient intake of protein because the amount eaten may not be sufficient to fulfill protein requirements. To calculate nutrient concentrations on an energy basis, the kilocalorie per kilogram of food should be known. This information may be obtained by the manufacturer or estimated by calculation (**Box 3**). The amount of grams of a nutrient per kilogram of food is determined and divided by the kilocalorie per kilogram of food (**Boxes 4** and **5**). This result gives the amount of nutrient per kilocalorie and is often multiplied by 100 or 1000 to give the amount per 100 kcal or 1000 kcal (1000 kcal = 1 Mcal). Energy-containing macronutrients are also sometimes expressed as the percentage of calories that contribute to the food (eg, 30% protein calories, 25% fat calories, and 45% carbohydrate calories) (see **Box 3**).

Product description (EU) and nutritional adequacy statement (US) state whether the food is nutritionally complete or complementary. In the United States, this statement must show the life stage for which the product is designed, the target animal species, and substantiation of the claim. AAFCO provides nutrient profiles and regulates pet food labeling for growth, reproduction, and adult maintenance, but not for senior/geriatric pets.[10,14] The claim must be substantiated by computer or laboratory analysis to be consistent with the AAFCO Dog/Cat Nutrient Profiles, and/or by feeding trials that comply with AAFCO guidelines.

If a label states a food is "complementary" or for "intermittent or supplemental use only," it is not a complete food and should usually not be fed as the sole diet. It may be acceptable if it is a veterinary therapeutic diet and is being used for a specific purpose (eg, dissolution of a specific type of urolithiasis), if it is being provided as a treat (see later discussion regarding treats), or if it is being used temporarily to stimulate an anorexic patient to eat.

Labels may include 1 of 2 statements regarding nutritional adequacy:

1. "[Name] is formulated to meet the nutritional levels established by the AAFCO Dog (or Cat) Food Nutrient Profiles for [life stage(s)]." (Calculated or chemical analysis of food.)

Box 3
Estimating the calorie content of a commercial food and determining the percentage of the energy from protein, fat, and carbohydrate

For example:

Label-guaranteed analysis:

Protein, min. 26%

Fat, min. 16%

Moisture, max. 12%

Ash, 5%

Crude fiber, 3%

Adding these percentages = 62%; then subtract 62% from 100% to determine an estimate of the amount of nonfiber carbohydrate (CHO), 100 − 62 = 38% CHO

To determine the calories of ME, multiply the major energy-providing foods (fiber does provide some energy, but ignore that for now) by their modified Atwater factors: 3.5 kcal/g each for protein and CHO; 8.5 kcal/g for fat:

Protein = 26 × 3.5 = 91

CHO = 38 × 3.5 = 133

Fat = 16 × 8.5 = 136

Add these = 360 kcal per 100 g.

Therefore, this diet would have 25% (91/360) of the calories derived from protein, 37% (133/360) from CHO, and 38% (136/360) from fat. Note that these are only estimates, because the nutrient guarantee will differ from typical analysis, and the Atwater factors may overestimate or underestimate true ME.

---

2. "Animal feeding tests using AAFCO procedures substantiate [Name] provides complete and balanced nutrition for [life stage(s)]." (Feeding trial analysis of food.)

   Feeding guidelines are directions for use, including recommended species, life stage, and recommended amounts. The feeding guidelines are based on average

---

Box 4
Comparing nutrients on an energy basis

If 2 diets contain different calorie density and the calories eaten are the same, the amount of nutrients consumed will be different; therefore, it may be useful to compare the nutrients in diets on an energy basis (eg, g protein/100 kcal). This can provide a better reflection of the animal's intake than the dry-matter basis. Example:

1. Diet A has 3500 kcal/kg as fed and diet B has 4500 kcal/g as fed; both diets have 10% moisture.

2. Both diets have 25% protein as fed.

3. On a dry-matter basis, the diets have 27.8% protein (25/0.90). On both diets, there are 250 g protein/kg of food (ie, 25% = 25 g/100 g = 250 g/kg).

4. However, if the patient consumes 1000 kcal per day, diet A will provide

   • 1000/3500 kcal × 250 g = 71.4 g protein eaten per day (ie, 71.4 g protein/1000 kcal).

5. If eating 1000 kcal on diet B

   • 1000/4500 kcal × 250 = 55.5 g protein eaten per day (ie, 55.5 g protein/1000 kcal).

> **Box 5**
> **Calculation of an estimated daily maintenance energy requirement**
>
> Maintenance energy requirements (MER), sometimes called daily energy requirements, are often determined based on resting energy requirements (RER). A commonly used equation for RER in kcal/day is: $70 \times$ body weight $(kg)^{0.75}$.
>
> Changes in the amount fed should be determined by body condition as the calculations are based on an "average" animal and should only be used as initial estimates.
>
> Feline MER (kcal/d)
>
>   Neutered adult: $1.2 \times$ RER
>
>   Intact adult: $1.4 \times$ RER
>
>   Active adult: $1.6 \times$ RER
>
>   Inactive/obese prone: $1.0 \times$ RER
>
>   Pregnancy: $1.6 \times$ RER at breeding, increase to 2 RER at queening
>
>   Lactation: $2–6 \times$ RER depending on the number of kittens
>
>   Growth: $2.5 \times$ RER
>
> The NRC recommends a different equation for MER for adult cats (kcal/d):
>
>   Lean cats: $100 \times$ body weight $(kg)^{0.67}$
>
>   Overweight cats: $130 \times$ body weight $(kg)^{0.40}$
>
> Either equation is likely adequate as long as changes in weight and BCS are monitored and food intake is appropriately adjusted.
>
> Canine MER (kcal/d)
>
>   Neutered adult: $1.6 \times$ RER
>
>   Intact adult: $1.8 \times$ RER
>
>   Inactive/obese prone: $1.4 \times$ RER
>
>   Weight loss: $1.0 \times$ RER
>
>   Work: $2–8 \times$ RER depending on duration and intensity
>
>   Pregnancy, first 42 days: $1.8 \times$ RER
>
>   Pregnancy, last 21 days, increase to: $3 \times$ RER
>
>   Lactation: $3–6 \times$ RER depending on number of puppies
>
>   Growth: $2–3 \times$ RER (decreased at around 4–6 months of age)

energy needs so may be too much or too little for an individual animal. They also assume that the pet food is the only food provided and do not account for extra treats or snacks. Veterinarians should discuss the variation among pets, the individuality of each pet's requirements, and the calories provided in treats and other added foods and teach owners about doing body condition scores (BCS; see Nutritional Assessment discussion later).

The caloric density of the food should be evaluated if the pet is below or above the desired BCS, or if the owner has to feed unusually large or small amounts to maintain a desired BCS. In the United States, the calorie content is or will be on the label; in other countries, it may be necessary to contact the company for this information.

Claims that the food will prevent, cure, or treat disease are not allowed by the FDA. Some of the other information provided on the label is of little practical value in assisting nutritional assessment. Because pet owners sometimes base their purchasing decisions on unregulated terms, such as "holistic," "human grade," or "premium," veterinarians and veterinary technicians must help them make informed decisions (**Table 1**). Although not a legal term, some pet food companies consider the use of the terms "premium" or "superpremium" to mean foods that have undergone extensive research, use a fixed nonvarying formula, contain high-quality ingredients, and often contain added ingredients, such as an antioxidant mix, which are thought to have health benefits for the pet. **Table 2** lists some Web sites that provide reliable information on nutrition for clinicians and for owners.

If the owner is feeding a homemade diet, it is highly possible that it is not complete and balanced (please also see the article in this issue by Parr and Remillard).[2] The practitioner should contact a veterinary nutritionist for advice in these cases. If raw meat diets are being fed, the owner should be counseled regarding potential health risks for the pet and any animal or person associated with the pet. Pathogenic bacteria may cause gastroenteritis and can be shed in the feces for up to 1 week after ingestion of contaminated raw meat. If a patient that has been fed a raw meat diet is hospitalized, the risk must be evaluated to hospital staff and other hospitalized animals. In addition, raw diets containing bones can be associated with dental damage and esophageal/gastrointestinal obstruction or perforation.[3] The practitioner should also be aware of the severe deficiencies of vegetarian diets if fed to cats, and it also should be considered carefully if a particular vegetarian diet is adequate for a dog as well.

NUTRITIONAL ASSESSMENT OF DOGS AND CATS

Incorporating nutritional assessment into patient care is critical for maintaining pets' health and their response to disease and injury. The World Small Animal Veterinary Association (WSAVA) has established an initiative for nutritional assessment to be the "5th vital sign" or fifth vital assessment (V5 or 5VA) after temperature, pulse, respiration, and pain assessment. Incorporating the screening evaluation as described in these guidelines as the fifth vital assessment in the standard physical examination requires little additional time and no cost.[15] Incorporating nutritional assessment and recommendations into the care of small animals also helps develop the partnership between the owner and veterinary health care team. Surveys show that owners have a desire to have information on nutrition and diet provided by the veterinary health care team.[16]

The American Animal Hospital Association (AAHA) published the AAHA Nutritional Assessment Guidelines for Dogs and Cats.[13] WSAVA then created a global version of the guidelines published as the Global Nutritional Assessment Guidelines.[16,17] Following the launch of the WSAVA's guidelines, the WSAVA Global Nutrition Committee (GNC) developed a suite of nutrition "tools" as a Toolkit (http://www.wsava.org/nutrition-toolkit).[15] These toolkits include practical aids for nutritional assessment, BCS charts (**Figs. 2** and **3**), and a video on assessing the body condition, muscle condition score chart (**Fig. 4**), guidelines for nutrition for hospitalized patients, average calorie recommendations for adult dogs and cats, and a nutritional assessment check sheet. There are also educational materials for pet owners, including guidelines for using information about nutrition from the Internet and picking the right diet. The tools are designed to help the veterinary health care team address nutrition and to advance the role of the team as the expert source of nutrition information.

What is a Nutritional Assessment?

Nutritional assessment includes consideration of animal-specific factors, diet-specific factors, feeding management, and environmental factors. Animal-specific factors

Table 1
Definitions of terms used in pet food marketing

Term	Definition	Comment
Organic	A feed or a specific ingredient within a formula feed that has been produced or handled in compliance with the requirements of the US Department of Agriculture (USDA) National Organic Program (AAFCO).	At least 95% of the ingredients need to be organic to have a USDA organic seal. Organic refers to the processing of a product, not the quality of the product.
Natural	A feed or ingredient derived solely from plant, animal, or mined sources, either in its unprocessed state or having been subject to physical processing, heat processing, rendering, purification, extraction, hydrolysis, enzymolysis, or fermentation, but not having been produced by or subject to a chemically synthetic process and not containing any additives or processing aids that are chemically synthetic except in amounts as might occur as unavoidable in good manufacturing practices.	Food will likely still require an antioxidant preservative to prevent fats from becoming rancid; added vitamins and minerals may be synthetic, and natural additives may not have been tested.
Hypoallergenic	No legal definition	Any ingredient, especially those containing whole (unhydrolyzed) protein, which an animal has previously been exposed to can potentially be allergenic. An allergic reaction is an abnormal response to a food or ingredient.
Human-grade food	A claim that something is "human-grade" or "human-quality" implies that the complete food is "edible" for people. The terms "human-grade" or "human-quality" have no legal definition.	Use is discouraged by AAFCO. If any portion of the food, processing, or handling is not suitable for foods for human consumption, then this claim is not appropriate.
Sustainable food	No legal definition—described as ensuring a better quality of life for everyone and the ability of society to be maintained over the long term (not compromising the ability of future generations to meet their needs)	Terminology likely to be used with different meanings by different companies and individuals.
Light, "lite" food, or low calorie	Dogs Dry food: 3100 kcal/kg as fed Canned food: 2500 kcal/kg as fed Cats Dry food: 3250 kcal/kg as fed Canned food: 2650 kcal/kg as fed (AAFCO)	If claim states "less calories," the percentage decrease compared with the similar product should be stated. Many pets will gain weight by being free-choice fed light foods.
Veterinarian approved	No legal definition	Ask which veterinarian and with what training?

(continued on next page)

Term	Definition	Comment
Table 1 (*continued*)		
Premium/ superpremium	No legal definition	Implies complete and balanced, use of a fixed recipe, good quality control, and possibly beneficial ingredients, but not regulated. May be higher in cost or sold only by veterinary practices or pet stores.
Holistic	No legal definition	May imply health benefits that do not exist.

include age, life stage, activity, and nutrient-sensitive disorders requiring specific dietary management (eg, chronic kidney disease, adverse reactions to food).

Diet-specific factors include the safety and appropriateness of the diet and include nutrient imbalances, spoilage, and contamination. The feeding of an unbalanced homemade diet or a poor-quality commercial diet would be considered at this point. Even a good nutritionally balanced diet may not be appropriate if it does not match the needs of an individual pet (eg, feeding an adult maintenance cat food to a kitten if the food is inadequate for growth).

Feeding factors include the frequency, timing, location, amount, and method of feeding. Information on feeding management includes overfeeding or underfeeding, feeding of treats, supplements, scavenging, and hunting. Environmental factors include the pet's housing, presence of other animals, access to the outdoors, and environmental enrichment.

Screening and Extended Evaluations

The initial nutritional assessment is a screening evaluation. If areas of concern are found during screening, an extended evaluation may be warranted. The screening evaluation should be performed for every pet at every visit as a part of routine history taking and physical examination. It includes a diet history, body weight, BCS, muscle condition score, and evaluation of the coat and teeth. The 9-point BCS scale (see **Figs. 2** and **3**) is used by the WSAVA. Body condition is determined using a combination of the visual appearance and palpation of the pet (eg, is there a waist apparent and palpation of the amount of fat cover over the ribs). The prevalence of obesity in the pet population makes performing and recording the BCS vitally important (for more on obesity, see the article by Linder and Mueller in this issue).

The BSC evaluates body fat, and it is possible for a pet to be overweight but still have muscle loss, especially in diabetic and other ill pets or the elderly. Muscle mass scoring systems are based on palpation of skeletal muscle over the skull, scapulae, spine, and pelvis (see **Fig. 4**). Acute and chronic disease may cause loss of muscle mass disproportionate to the loss of fat due to the cytokine and neurohormonal effects on metabolism. An example that is commonly seen in practice is the diabetic cat, which appears thin and bony along its top line but has retained its inguinal fat pad.

Dietary and Feeding Management Plan

Following the nutritional assessment, the owner should be provided with a dietary recommendation and feeding management plan written on a discharge sheet along with other any instructions (eg, for medications). This feeding management plan can

Table 2
Some of the professional organizations and Web sites providing reliable nutrition advice

Organization	Description or Objectives	Web site
American Academy of Veterinary Nutrition	An international association of veterinarians and animal scientists with a common interest in animal nutrition as it relates to animal health. Does not require examination to join; does require evidence of working in the area of animal nutrition.	www.aavn.org
American College of Veterinary Nutrition	The primary objectives are to advance the specialty area of veterinary nutrition and increase the competence of those who practice in this field by establishing requirements for certification in veterinary nutrition, encouraging continuing professional education, promoting research, and enhancing the dissemination of new knowledge of veterinary nutrition through didactic teaching and postgraduate programs. Members have done a residency in veterinary nutrition and passed a rigorous examination to qualify.	www.acvn.org
European Society of Veterinary and Comparative Nutrition	Objectives: to generate interest, stimulate research, and disseminate knowledge in veterinary nutrition and nutrition-related diseases, to promote pregraduate and postgraduate education in veterinary nutrition, to stimulate the application of clinical nutrition in veterinary schools by cooperation between nutritionists and clinicians, and to cooperate with other societies with related interests.	www.esvcn.com
European College of Comparative Veterinary Nutrition	A body of veterinarians specialized in nutrition. ECVCN is member of the European Board of Veterinary Specialisation. To be accepted to the examinations to become a Diplomate of the ECVCN, candidates have to be veterinarians and need to have experience in practical nutrition with healthy and sick animals besides having performed research in nutrition.	Within www.esvcn.com Web site
WSAVA and the GNC	An association of associations. Its membership is made up of veterinary organizations from all over the world, which are concerned with companion animals. Within the organization is the GNC, which is dedicated to improving knowledge and practice of nutrition. It developed global nutrition guidelines, the goal of which is to help the veterinary health care team and pet owners ensure that dogs and cats are on an optimal nutrition plan tailored to the needs of the individual dog or cat. These guidelines have now been expanded into a practitioner and owner-friendly toolkit on the Web site.	www.wsava.org

be from the WSAVA Nutritional Assessment check sheet, or a short section on a discharge sheet recommending what, how much, and how often to feed. If no change is recommended, the owners should be advised that the current diet is adequate to reinforce good habits.

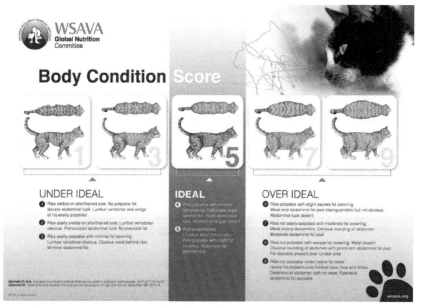

Fig. 2. Feline BCS. (*Courtesy of* World Small Animal Veterinary Association, Ontario, Canada; with permission.)

The nutritional recommendation depends on whether the animal is healthy or ill and if it is to be hospitalized. Some factors that need to be considered include the animal's energy (calorie) needs, protein requirements, special dietary needs for disease, nutrient losses via diarrhea, urine (eg, proteinuria or glucosuria), or drains.

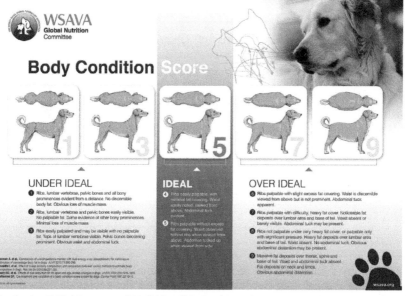

Fig. 3. Canine BCS. (*Courtesy of* World Small Animal Veterinary Association, Ontario, Canada; with permission.)

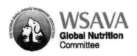

Muscle Condition Score

Muscle condition score is assessed by visualization and palpation of the spine, scapulae, skull, and wings of the ilia. Muscle loss is typically first noted in the epaxial muscles on each side of the spine; muscle loss at other sites can be more variable. Muscle condition score is graded as normal, mild loss, moderate loss, or severe loss. Note that animals can have significant muscle loss if they are overweight (body condition score > 5). Conversely, animals can have a low body condition score (< 4) but have minimal muscle loss. Therefore, assessing both body condition score and muscle condition score on every animal at every visit is important. Palpation is especially important when muscle loss is mild and in animals that are overweight. An example of each score is shown below.

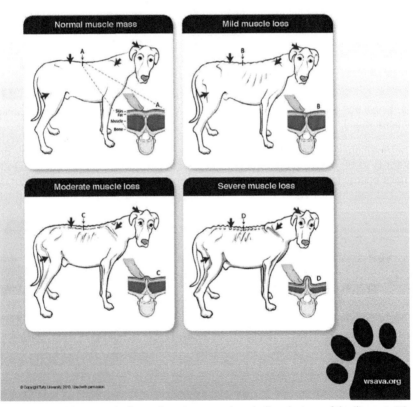

Fig. 4. Canine MCS. *Arrows* indicate the spine, scapulae, skull and wings of the ilium. *A–D* indicate increasing severity of muscle loss. (*Courtesy of* World Small Animal Veterinary Association, Ontario, Canada; with permission.)

Although calorie requirements for cats or dogs can vary up to 50% from the estimated amount, the amount should be calculated as a starting point. Average maintenance or daily energy requirements (which are equivalent) for adult dogs and cats of healthy body condition may be calculated (see **Box 4**) or found on the WSAVA GNC Toolkit.[15] Working or agility dogs often need more than these estimates and the adult calculations should not be used for reproducing or growing pets, because they have much higher needs.

The owner's preferences should also be considered (eg, if they work full time, feeding multiple times per day may not be feasible). In addition to the primary diet, the practitioner should evaluate other sources of nutrients (eg, treats, table food, supplements, food used for administering medication, chew toys [eg, rawhide]). Owners often do not consider food used for administering medication as a "treat" and may not mention it. Although treats and snacks are part of the owner's relationship with the pet, they should be taken into account and advice given for appropriate treats. Asking an owner to stop feeding treats may result in poor compliance; it is better to give advice that will work for the owner. For adult animals, if snacks and treats comprise 10% or less of the total calories, they are not liable to significantly unbalance a good-quality complete diet.

A nutritional evaluation and diet recommendation should be made at every veterinary visit. Tools provided in the WSAVA Toolkit will be useful when developing or expanding the nutritional focus in a veterinary practice.

INTEGRATING NUTRITIONAL ASSESSMENTS INTO A BUSY GENERAL PRACTICE

Trying to integrate anything new into a busy practice can be daunting; however, because the need is great, it is well worth the effort. The following plan was used to implement the nutritional guidelines into a busy practice.

Awareness and Education (Secure Staff Support)

Initial awareness initiated at one of the weekly doctors' meetings, where the doctors discussed the new nutritional assessment guidelines, recognized that consistent and confident recommendations often were not given even though clients desired the information, and many of the patients were in obvious need. Once agreement was established that nutrition was important, exposure to the materials in the WSAVA GNC Toolkit[15] provided them with an increased confidence that they had the necessary tools to move forward with this new process. Paramount to acceptance was the understanding that appropriate nutrition and advice were in the best interest of the patient.

In addition, the culture of the practice was discussed with knowledge that the entire team of support individuals would need to think this was important to the patient and the owner. To this end, several of the monthly staff meetings were dedicated to education regarding the many benefits of appropriate nutrition as well as the myths and health hazards of inappropriate nutrition.

Initiation

To facilitate incorporation into the everyday examination, templates were created to include what was thought to be the most important aspects of nutritional assessment (**Fig. 5**). Most of this was placed into the history portion or the subjective ("S") portion of a problem-oriented record-keeping system (subjective, objective, assessment, and plan or SOAP record-keeping).

Incorporation into the history and examination template better assured that the appropriate questions were asked and an assessment made. This template attempted to encompass what was needed for the "screening evaluation" and most of these questions should have been asked anyway for any wellness or nonwell examination.

The examination "O" portion of the template incorporated BCS and muscle condition scores (MCS) as well as current and previous weights. The assessment (A) portion of the

The Parkway Veterinary Hospital
3 S.W. Monroe Pkwy, Suite Y
Lake Oswego, OR
(503) 636-2102
02/04/2013

Physical Exam Findings:
Cat Fake's physical examination is below.

Her weight today is:
Previous Weight:
Body Condition Score (1-9):
(1 - emaciated, 5 - ideal, 9 - grossly obese)

Temperature:

Attitude and Appearance:
Hydration Level:
Eyes, Ears, Nose, Throat:
Capillary Refill Time/Mucous Membranes:
Oral exam/Calculus level (0-4):

Cardiovascular/Heartrate:
Pulmonary/Respiratory:

Peripheral Lymph nodes:
Abdominal Palpation:
Urogenital:
Anal glands and rectum:

Skin/Integument and Nails:
Musculoskeletal/Neurologic function:
Muscle Condition Score (1-4):
(4 - normal, 2 - mild muscle wasting, 1 - severe muscle wasting)
Pain Score (0-5):

Assessment:
Nutritional Assessment:

RECOMMENDATIONS:
Nutritional Recommendation(s):

Date Created: 02/04/2013 Time: 08:43:22 PM

Fig. 5. Example of a nutritional assessment template used in practice.

template incorporated the question on nutritional assessment of current diet, whereas the treatment plan (P) incorporated the nutritional recommendation. See **Fig. 5** for an example of an examination template incorporating nutritional assessments.

In this practice, there were no defaults, as it was thought that a blank portion of a physical examination would indicate not examined or assessed and would not be as misleading as a default to "normal" or "good."

In addition, many of the tools and handouts from the WSAVA GNC Toolkit were copied and provided to clients, giving them industry-neutral information regarding nutrition.[15]

Monitor and Review

Several months after initiation of the guidelines, critical reviews of the process of nutritional assessment during examinations were initiated. Alternatively, they can be reviewed continuously and updated and/or modified as needed, based on staff feedback. For example, revised BCS and MCS diagrams were introduced and discussed during doctor meetings. Also, the "examination" template containing much of the nutritional assessment verbiage could be modified if needed.

Comments

Adding the Nutritional Assessment principles to a standard examination and creating a template absolutely improved the consistency of the total examination for the patients. This addition minimized missed lesions or questions for any disease or wellness examination. It was common for the questions to generate discussions with clients about nutrition that would not have taken place otherwise. It did add some time to the examinations, but by making this the responsibility of the entire practice team (which they agreed was in the best interest of the patient), much of this was accomplished before the doctor entered the room. Also, the entire staff agreed that better wellness care and prevention are now being provided than previously.

NUTRITION MYTHS AND MISCONCEPTIONS

There is a myriad of "information" about nutrition available to owners in books and on Web sites. Some of this information is accurate and evidence-based; much of it is opinion without factual basis. Owners may be feeding an unconventional diet (eg, an unbalanced homemade diet or an unbalanced commercial diet recommended by a Web site). A good dietary history (see above) will reveal this and allow the clinician the opportunity of discussing the owner's choices. Most owners do want nutrition information from the health care team.

Some of the myths and misconceptions that lead owners to feed an unconventional diet are discussed.

Myth: Large-Breed Puppies Should Be Fed an Adult Maintenance Diet to Prevent Developmental Orthopedic Disease

Decreasing the risk of developmental orthopedic disease in large-breed puppies does involve restricted energy intake to keep puppies from growing too rapidly or becoming fat; however, it may be preferable to feed a puppy diet designed for large-breed puppies. Some diets formulated for adult dogs may be too low in protein and possibly too low in calcium and phosphorus or have an incorrect calcium:phosphorus ratio. The veterinarian should check that the nutrient amounts in the diet meet the requirements for growth. The diets for growth should not be supplemented with additional calcium or other minerals. Once the large-breed puppy reaches adult size, they may be changed to an adult maintenance diet.[18]

Myth: Dry Diets Cause Gastric Dilation Volvulus

Studies on nutritional risks for gastric dilation volvulus (GDV) include dry food that has oil or fat among the first 4 ingredients, and that moistening the food increased the risk. Large food particles (>30 mm) decrease the risk.[19] In one study, feeding a single food type, such as dry or canned, increased the risk, whereas adding canned food or table scraps to a commercial dry diet reduced the risk.[20] Feeding once a day and rapid ingestion of food were also noted as risk factors.[20] It appears that feeding from a height, previously recommended as a preventative measure, may also increase the risk of GDV.[21] It should be noted that many studies have been undertaken to evaluate the role of diet in GDV and the findings are not always consistent; however, no studies have unequivocally documented a link between feeding dry food and an increased risk of GDV.

Myth: Fasting Is an Effect Method for Weight Loss

Fasting will result in weight loss; however, fasting appears to slow down the metabolic rate more than gradual weight loss. This slowed metabolism continues after "normal" eating resumes, making it easier for the animal to regain the weight. Fasting also causes a greater loss of lean body mass (eg, muscles) than does a low-calorie diet. The decrease in lean body mass contributes to the lower metabolic rate.[22] Cats that are fasted or lose weight too quickly can develop hepatic lipidosis.[23]

Myth: Feeding Brewer's Yeast, or Onions, or Garlic, Prevents Fleas

Feeding brewer's yeast supplies some B vitamins, but does nothing for flea prevention.[24] Adding too much yeast abruptly to a diet may cause flatulence. There is no evidence that feeding onions and garlic prevents fleas, and they contain several sulfur compounds (eg, allium in garlic) that can cause red blood cell lysis because of the formation of Heinz bodies.[25–27]

Myth: Dogs Should Have Bones to Eat/Chew

Bones are often fed to dogs as a source of dietary calcium and/or to clean their teeth (or simply because they enjoy them). Giving whole bones is an erratic and generally inadequate way of adding calcium to the diet, although ground bone meal does provide calcium and may be used in some diets. Bones will often pass through the gastrointestinal tract without problems, but occasionally a fragment may obstruct or perforate the bowel, causing rapid death. Eating bones can also cause constipation.[3] Large beef bones that can be chewed without splintering (ie, not swallowed) can be enjoyable for dogs. They may help to prevent dental tartar, although they can also cause teeth to break and one study showed evidence of periodontitis in wild dogs eating a "natural" diet, even though only mild calculus deposits were found.[28] In a study on feral cats eating a "wild natural" diet and domestic cats being fed commercial food, there was no difference in the prevalence of periodontitis, although dental calculus scores were higher in the domestic cats.[29] Another study showed an increased risk of oral health problems in dogs and cats fed a homemade diet compared with those fed commercial food.[30]

Myth: Raw Diets Are Better Because They Are More Natural

Raw diets often contain bacteria and may be contaminated with pathogenic organisms such as salmonella, parasites, and protozoa. Handling raw diets can pose a health hazard to humans, because there is an increased risk of exposure to the same pathogens. Finally, such diets may not to be nutritionally balanced.[3,31,32] For more information, see the article by Parr and Remillard in this issue.

Myth: Gluten-Free Diets Are Healthier for Dogs and Cats

Only 1% to 1.5% of people have celiac disease (an adverse reaction to the gluten in wheat products),[33] but gluten-free diets have become a popular concept recently and this has spilled over into the pet food area as well. Such wheat/gluten sensitivities appear to be uncommon in pets, although the true prevalence is unknown. Some Irish setters do appear to be sensitive to gluten.[34] In 330 dogs of various breeds with a diagnosis of adverse reaction to food, the most common allergenic ingredients were beef, dairy, and chicken, with wheat the fourth listed ingredient.[35] Only 4 and 3 of 56 cats with adverse reactions to food had a reaction to corn/corn gluten and wheat, respectively. The most common reactions in cats were to beef, dairy, fish, and chicken.[35] To prove an adverse reaction to food, a food elimination and challenge trial should be done; without the challenge, the reason for a response to diet change is speculative. Gluten is a very high-quality protein and is highly digestible; it appears to be an acceptable ingredient for most pets.[36]

Myth: Senior Dogs and Cats Should Be Fed a Low-Protein Diet to Prevent Kidney Disease

This misconception is due to old literature based on rodent studies and has since been disproven. The protein content in a food does not appear to have a causal effect in chronic kidney disease. Even in the treatment of kidney disease, phosphorous restriction is likely more important than limiting protein intake. Pets may need more high-quality, highly digestible protein as they age because sarcopenia (muscle loss) is associated with aging.[37,38]

Myth: By-Products Are Poor Quality Ingredients

Meat and poultry by-products or secondary products are unused portions of food that come from clean and healthy food animals used for human consumption. Meat by-products are defined by AAFCO[7] as "The non-rendered, clean parts, other than meat derived from slaughtered mammals. It includes, but is not limited to, lungs, spleen, kidneys, brain, liver, blood, bone, partially defatted low temperature fatty tissue and stomachs and intestines freed from their contents. It does not include hair, horns, teeth and hoofs," and poultry by-products "must consist of non-rendered clean parts of carcasses of slaughtered poultry such as heads, feet, viscera, free from fecal content and foreign matter except in such trace amounts as might occur unavoidably in good factory practice." By-products do not include the unwanted waste parts, including gastrointestinal contents, horns, teeth, hooves, and diseased or cancerous animal parts. By-products can be an excellent and healthy source of nutrition.[7,39]

Myth: Feeding Dry Food to Cats Causes Diabetes Mellitus Because of the High-Carbohydrate Content

Cats are obligate carnivores and are less efficient than some other mammals at metabolizing large amounts of dietary carbohydrates.[40,41] In one study on macronutrient selection, the cats chose a low-carbohydrate diet, although they are capable of digesting carbohydrates[42,43] and many cats do prefer dry to canned diets. Overweight cats did show insulin resistance, especially when fed a very high-carbohydrate, low-protein diet,[44] but the profile of this diet is not consistent with most commercial cat foods. Carbohydrates, such as found in most dry cat foods, do not induce hyperglycemia in healthy cats. Different grains and the processing of the grains can also affect the blood glucose and insulin responses.[45,46] Risk factor for type 2 diabetes in cats has been reported to include indoor confinement, low physical activity,[47] and neutering,[48] but not the proportion of dry diet or high dietary carbohydrates. Increased body fat (overweight or obese body condition) is more likely than the type of diet to induce a prediabetic condition.[49,50]

There is little question that once a cat develops diabetes mellitus, feeding a high-protein, low-carbohydrate diet will increase the chance of remission (no longer dependent on exogenous insulin).

SUMMARY

Diet may help treat, or decrease the risk of, disease, or cause it if there are problems with the food or feeding management. To evaluate pet foods, practitioners should be aware of what nutrient requirements have been used to formulate the diet and if it has been tested by computer, chemical analysis, and/or feeding trials. The nutrient analysis on pet foods may be used to compare foods if they are compared on an energy or dry-matter basis. The food should state on the label if it is complete and balanced and what species and life stage it is designed to feed. When recommending a diet to the owner, the practitioner should ensure that it is complete and balanced, has adequate digestibility, and is safe. High-quality diets may have ingredients with added health benefits.

A screening nutritional assessment should be performed for every pet at every veterinary visit. This screening nutritional assessment will allow the health care team to ensure that good diet and feeding management practices are being used. It is possible and beneficial to incorporate nutritional assessment into a busy practice and adds value for pets, owners, and staff.

Myths and misconceptions about nutrition abound in veterinary medicine. The practitioner should seek evidence-based research rather than anecdotes to find information about nutrition.

REFERENCES

1. Buffington T, Holloway C, Abood S. Chapter 5 Clinical dietetics. In: Manual of veterinary dietetics. St Louis (MO): Elsevier Saunders; 2004. p. 49–142.
2. Stockman J, Fascetti AJ, Kass PH, et al. Evaluation of recipes of home-prepared maintenance diets for dogs. Timely Topics in Nutrition. J Am Vet Med Assoc 2013;242(11):1500–5.
3. Freeman LM, Chandler ML, Hamper BA, et al. Current knowledge about the risks and benefits of raw meat-based diets for dogs and cats. J Am Vet Med Assoc 2013;243(11):1549–58.
4. Rumbeiha W, Morrison J. A review of class I and class II pet food recalls involving chemical contaminants from 1996 to 2008. J Med Toxicol 2011;7:60–6.
5. Available at: www.vin.com/doc/?id=5139625. Accessed November 1, 2013.
6. Buffington T, Holloway C, Abood S. Chapter 4 Diet and diet feeding factors. In: Manual of veterinary dietetics. St Louis (MO): Elsevier Saunders; 2004. p. 39–48.
7. Association of American Feed Control Officials, Inc. 2013 Official publication. Oxford (IN): Association of American Feed Control Officials, Inc; 2011. Available at: www.aafco.org.
8. National Research Council (NRC). Nutrient requirements of dogs and cats. Washington, DC: National Academy Press; 2006.
9. FEDIAF Nutritional guidelines cats and dogs. Available at: www.fediaf.org/self-regulation/nutrition/. Accessed November 3, 2013.
10. Burger IH, Thompson A. Reading a petfood label. In: Will JM, Simpson KW, editors. The Waltham book of clinical nutrition of the dog and cat. Oxford (England): Pergammon; 1994. p. 15–24.
11. Kienzle EI, Schrag I, Butterwick R, et al. Calculations of gross energy in pet foods; do we have the right values for heat of combustion. J Nutr 2002;132:1799S–800S.
12. Laflamme DP. Determining metabolizable energy content in commercial pet foods. J Anim Physiol Anim Nutr (Berl) 2001;85:222–30.

13. Baldwin K, Bartges J, Buffington T, et al. AAHA nutritional assessment guidelines for dogs and cats. J Am Anim Hosp Assoc 2010;46(4):285–96.
14. Delaney SJ, Fascetti AJ. Using pet food labels and product guides. In: Fascetti AJ, Delaney SJ, editors. Applied veterinary clinical nutrition. Chichester (England): Wiley-Blackwell; 2012. p. 69–74.
15. Available at: www.WSAVA.org. Accessed November 5, 2013.
16. American Animal Hospital Association. Quantifying opportunities available by increasing compliance rates. The path to high-quality care: practical tips for improving compliance. Lakewood (CO): American Animal Hospital Association; 2003. p. 385–96.
17. WSAVA Nutritional Assessment Guidelines Task Force Members, Freeman L, Becvarova I, et al. WSAVA Nutritional Assessment Guidelines. J Small Anim Pract 2011;52(7):385–96.
18. Lauten SD. Nutritional risks to large-breed dogs: from weaning to the geriatric years. Vet Clin North Am Small Anim Pract 2006;36(6):1324–60.
19. Theyse LF, van de Brom WE, Slujis FJ. Small size of food particles and age as risk factors for gastric dilatation volvulus in Great Danes. Vet Rec 1998;143(2):48–50.
20. Glickman LT, Glickman NW, Schellenberg DB, et al. Risk factors for the gastric dilatation-volvulus syndrome in practitioner/owner case-control study. J Am Anim Hosp Assoc 1997;33(3):197–204.
21. Raghavan M, Glickman NW, Glickman L. The effect of ingredients in dry dog foods on the risk of gastric dilatation-volvulus in dogs. J Am Anim Hosp Assoc 2006;42(1):28–36.
22. Laflamme DP, Kuhlman G. The effect of weight loss regimen on subsequent weight maintenance in dogs. Nutr Res 1995;15:1019–28.
23. Center S. Hepatic lipidosis, glucocorticoid hepatopathy, vacuolar hepatopathy, storage disorders, amyloidosis, and iron toxicity. In: Guilford WG, Center SA, Strombeck DR, et al, editors. Strombeck's small animal gastroenterology. 3rd edition. Philadelphia: WB Saunders; 1996. p. 766–801.
24. Baker NF, Farve T. Failure of brewer's yeast as a repellent to fleas on dogs. J Am Vet Med Assoc 1983;183(2):212–4.
25. Tang X, Xia Z, Yu J. An experimental study of hemolysis induced by onion (Allium cepa) poisoning in dogs. J Vet Pharmacol Ther 2008;31(2):143–9.
26. National Research Council. Garlic. In: National Research Council, editor. Safety of dietary supplements for horses dogs and cats. Washington, DC: The Academy Press; 2009. p. 135–68.
27. Freeman LM, Michel KE. Evaluation of raw food diets for dogs. J Am Vet Med Assoc 2001;218(5):705–9.
28. Steenkamp G, Gorrel C. Oral and dental conditions in adult African wild dog skulls: a preliminary report. J Vet Dent 1999;16(2):65–8.
29. Clarke DE, Cameron A. Relationship between diet, dental calculus and periodontal disease in domestic and feral cats in Australia. Aust Vet J 1998;76(10):690–3.
30. Buckley C, Colyer A, Slrywanek M, et al. The impact of home prepared diets and home oral hygiene on oral health in cats and dogs. Br J Nutr 2011;106:S24–7.
31. Schlesinger DP, Joffe DJ. Raw food diets in companion animals: a critical review. Can Vet J 2011;52(1):50–4.
32. Joffe DJ, Schlesinger DP. Preliminary assessment of the risk of Salmonella infection in dogs fed raw chicken diets. Can Vet J 2002;43:441–2.
33. Susanna A, Elisa G, Fausto M, et al. Mass population screening for celiac disease in children: the experience in Republic of San Marino from 1993 to 2009. J Pediatr 2013;39(1):67–70.

34. Guilford WG. Adverse reactions to food. In: Guilford WG, Center SA, Strombeck DR, et al, editors. Strombeck's small animal gastroenterology. 3rd edition. Philadelphia: WB Saunders; 1996. p. 436–50.

35. Roudebush P. Ingredients and foods associated with adverse reactions in dogs and cats. Vet Dermatol 2013;24:292–4.

36. Case LM, Daristotle L, Hayek MG, et al. Nutrient content of pet foods. In: Canine and feline nutrition. 3rd edition. Maryland Heights (MO): Mosby Elsevier; 2011. p. 141–62.

37. Laflamme DP. Pet food safety: dietary protein. Top Companion Anim Med 2008; 23(3):154–7.

38. Elliott DA. Nutritional management of chronic kidney disease in dogs and cats. Vet Clin North Am Small Anim Pract 2006;36(6):1377–84.

39. Wortinger A. Nutritional myths. J Am Anim Hosp Assoc 2005;41(4):273–6.

40. Buffington CA. Dry foods and risk of disease in cats. Can Vet J 2008;49(6): 561–3.

41. Hewson-Hughes A, Gilham MS, Upton S, et al. Postprandial glucose and insulin profiles following a glucose-loaded meal in cats and dogs. Br J Nutr 2011; 106(Suppl 1):S101–4.

42. Hewson-Hughes AK, Hewson-Hughes VL, Colyer A, et al. Consistent proportional macronutrient intake selected by adult domestic cats (Felis catus) despite variations in macronutrient and moisture content of foods offered. J Comp Physiol B 2013;183:525–36.

43. Martin GJ, Rand JS. Food intake and blood glucose in normal and diabetic cats fed ad libitum. J Feline Med Surg 1999;1:241–51.

44. Hoenig M, Thomaseth K, Waldron M, et al. Fatty acid turnover, substrate oxidation, and heat production in lean and obese cats during the euglycemic hyperinsulinemic clamp. Domest Anim Endocrinol 2007;4:329–98.

45. Appleton DJ, Rand JS, Sunvold GD, et al. Dietary carbohydrate source affects glucose concentrations, insulin secretion and food intake in overweight cats. Nutr Res 2004;24:447–67.

46. de-Oliveira LD, Carciofi AC, Oliveira CC, et al. Effects of six carbohydrate sources on diet digestibility and postprandial glucose and insulin responses in cats. J Anim Sci 2008;86:2237–46.

47. Slingerland LI, Fazilova VV, Plantinga EA, et al. Indoor confinement and physical activity rather than the proportion of dry food are risk factors in the development of feline type 2 diabetes mellitus. Vet J 2007;179(2):247–53.

48. Backus RC, Cave NJ, Keisler DH. Gonadectomy and high dietary fat but not high dietary carbohydrate induce gains in body and fat of domestic cats. Br J Nutr 2007;98:641–50.

49. Backus RC, Cave NJ, Ganjam VK, et al. Age and body weight effects on glucose and insulin tolerance in colony cats maintained since weaning on high dietary carbohydrate. J Anim Physiol Anim Nutr (Berl) 2010;94(6):318–28.

50. Hoenig M, Thomaseth K, Waldron M, et al. Insulin sensitivity, fat distribution, and adipocytokine response to different diets in lean and obese cats before and after weight loss. Am J Physiol Regul Integr Comp Physiol 2007;292(1):R227–34.

Handling Alternative Dietary Requests from Pet Owners

Jacqueline M. Parr, DVM, MSc[a,b,*],
Rebecca L. Remillard, PhD, DVM[c,d,e]

KEYWORDS

- Alternative diets • Unconventional diets • Homemade diets (cooked, raw)
- Commercial pet foods • Nutritional adequacy • Nutritional assessment

KEY POINTS

- We have proposed the use of the term "alternative" to encompass the wide variety of dietary options available to pet owners that are not viewed as conventional dry (ie, kibble) or canned (ie, wet) foods produced on a large commercial scale.
- There is *no way* a practitioner can keep up with the vast number of pet food products available on the market, so more likely than not, clients will be naming pet foods and feeding product combinations that are *unfamiliar to them*.
- Our approach to categorizing alternative diets is based on the nutritional adequacy of these dietary options, and we have developed three categories of nutritional adequacy that then dictate whether or not further evaluation is needed on the part of the practitioner.
- Patients will be at risk for nutrition-related diseases if fed a nutritionally incomplete or improperly balanced diet long term.
- To remain competitive, practitioners must consider raising their level of nutritional competency or incorporating the specialty of nutrition, through consultants if needed, into their practice to meet the growing client demand for dietary information specific to their pet.

Funding Sources: None.
Conflict of Interest: On Parr Nutrition, Inc (J.M. Parr); Veterinary Nutritional Consultations, Inc and www.PetDiets.com (R.L. Remillard).

[a] Clinical Nutrition Service, Department of Clinical Studies, Ontario Veterinary College, University of Guelph, 50 Stone Road West, Guelph, Ontario N1G 2W1, Canada; [b] On Parr Nutrition, Inc, Guelph, ON N1G4S7, Canada; [c] Nutrition Service, Small and Large Animal Nutrition, Molecular Biomedical Science Department, College of Veterinary Medicine, North Carolina State University, 1052 William Moore Drive, Raleigh, NC 27607, USA; [d] Veterinary Nutritional Consultations, Inc, 1002 Capps Farm Road, Hollister, NC 27844, USA; [e] Consultant Rayne Clinical Nutrition LLC, Po Box 481813, Kansas City, MO 64148, USA
* Corresponding author. Clinical Nutrition Service, Department of Clinical Studies, Ontario Veterinary College, University of Guelph, 50 Stone Road West, Guelph, Ontario N1G 2W1, Canada.
E-mail address: parr@uoguelph.ca

Vet Clin Small Anim 44 (2014) 667–688
http://dx.doi.org/10.1016/j.cvsm.2014.03.006
0195-5616/14/$ – see front matter © 2014 Elsevier Inc. All rights reserved.

vetsmall.theclinics.com

INTRODUCTION

Although the exact timing and location of the first domesticated dogs remains a source of debate, dogs have been living in close proximity with humans for at least the past 10,000 years.[1] In fact, dogs were likely the first animals to become domesticated, and genetic adaptation to efficient starch digestion was a key point in the domestication of dogs from wolves.[1] Despite this lengthy proximity to humans, foods specifically designed for dogs have been in use for only the past 150 years.[2,3]

The first dog biscuit, now known as "Milk-Bone," was produced and sold in 1860 by James Spratt, an American living in London, England.[2,3] The first canned dog food was produced in Illinois in 1922 called "Ken-L-Ration."[2,3] Notably, in the early 1940s, canned pet food represented more than 90% of manufactured pet food.[2,3] However, World War II changed the course of the commercial pet food industry in North America when the government instituted the rationing of meat and the metal used for packaging canned foods for the war effort.[2,3] In the mid-1940s, dry pet foods had taken over the lion's share of the market, representing 85% of pet foods sold.[2] For many pet owners and veterinarians alike, it may come as a surprise that manufacturing of extruded kibble for dogs and cats was first introduced in the late 1950s by Purina, making this technology less than 60 years old.[2,3]

The reason for taking a moment to relive a bit of pet food industry history is to illustrate that before 100 years ago, what we consider to be the traditional landscape of the pet food industry nowadays did not even exist. In fact, what are considered to be "unconventional" diets for pets nowadays are what pets were consuming more than 100 years ago (albeit in a much less complete and balanced fashion). Before these commercial products, dogs were fed homemade diets using leftovers and table scraps, and they scavenged our garbage or hunted their own food. Thus, over the long history of dogs' close association with humans, feeding what we consider today to be the norm, a commercially made dry or canned product, is a recent event.

Today, commercial pet foods are a mainstay of dog and cat nutrition. No doubt the vast majority of dogs and cats in the United States and Canada are fed a commercially made product and this is currently considered the norm. A plethora of diets are manufactured in North America for dogs and cats, typically in the form of dry (ie, kibble) or wet (ie, canned) foods. A 2008 survey in the United States and Australia revealed more than 90% of dogs and approximately 99% of cats receive at least half of their dietary intake from a commercially made pet food.[4] Dry kibble is most commonly fed to dogs and cats are more likely to receive wet foods than dogs.[4]

What Is a "Conventional" Versus an "Unconventional" Diet?

If we consider commercially made pet foods to be "conventional" diets, then "unconventional" diets have typically been defined as homemade diets, with either cooked or raw ingredients that pet owners prepare themselves. In the same 2008 survey, approximately 15% of cats and 30% of dogs in the United States and Australia consumed a combination of "unconventional" (eg, homemade diets, table scraps, and/or raw meat and bones) and commercial pet foods.[4] However, over the past decade, the distinct line between "unconventional" and "conventional" diets has become blurred with the introduction of products that resemble "homemade" but are produced on a large commercial scale. Commercialization of "unconventional" diets originally started with packaged raw food diets and has progressed to include products resembling TV dinners (ie, just heat and serve) and meal "helpers" (eg, Hamburger Helper for pets). Not only has the number of dietary options increased, but the market locations where these products are available span across grocery stores, mass merchandisers, pet specialty stores, and veterinary clinics.

This brings into question the use of the terms "conventional" versus "unconventional." The American Animal Hospital Association (AAHA)[5] and World Small Animal Veterinary Association (WSAVA)[6] have developed nutritional assessment guidelines (www.everypeteverytime.com/nutrition-assessment.html) for all patients at every visit. These guidelines have a list of nutrition-related risk factors by which if any one of the risk factors is recognized during the initial screening of a patient, a more thorough examination of the patient, diet, and method of feeding is recommended. One of the nutritional risk factors listed is feeding an "unconventional diet (eg, raw, homemade, vegetarian, unfamiliar)".[6] *We suggest this terminology may not be sufficiently helpful to the practitioner.*

But what is a "conventional" versus an "unconventional" diet? Other than suggesting "raw, homemade, and vegetarian diets" are "unconventional," neither AAHA nor WSAVA offer a description of a "conventional" versus "unconventional" diet.[5,6] The word "conventional" is a subjective adjective defined as, "in accordance with what is generally done or believed."[7] Synonyms are normal, standard, ordinary, usual, traditional, typical, and common.[7] One might assume based on the billions of dollars spent annually that kibble, followed by canned foods, with a nutritional claim of complete and balanced, made by a "major" pet food company, are the "conventional" diets. AAHA and the WSAVA received support from Hill's Pet Nutrition, Nestlé Purina Pet Care, Procter & Gamble Pet Care, and Royal Canin, and each manufacturer had an industry representative on the Global Nutrition Committee, which may have also influenced the thinking on what is or is not a "conventional" pet food product.

If the previous definition of "conventional" holds true, "unconventional" diets are considered to be any deviation from feeding a commercially manufactured diet that is intended to be the sole source of nutrition for dogs and cats. Unfortunately, this distinction is unlikely to hold true in the near future (and perhaps even at present) because of the number and variety of commercially made pet food products available to pet owners today. The most recent American Pet Products Association (APPA) National Pet Owner Survey indicated that the feeding practices of pet owners are highly varied and not limited to one type of pet food, as illustrated by the significant percentage of owners feeding human, frozen, raw, and vegetarian food products, as shown in **Table 1**.[8] Therefore, describing a diet risk factor as "unconventional" is not sufficiently discerning to help practitioners identify those pets eating a nutritionally inadequate diet and therefore at risk for a nutrition-related disease.

New Thinking: "Alternative" Diets

We would like to propose the use of the term "alternative" to encompass the dietary options available to pet owners today that are not commercially manufactured kibble or canned foods with a nutritional claim of complete and balanced. "Alternative" can be defined as "something different from, and able to serve as a substitute for, or another possibility."[9] In many instances, an alternative dietary product can be complete and balanced, serve as the sole source of nutrition, and be a reliable substitute for commercial kibble or canned foods; however, the nutritional adequacy of alternative diets is not as readily apparent as with commercially manufactured kibble or canned foods.

More and more pet owners desire conversations regarding alternative diets with their veterinarians. If pet owner concerns about alternative diets are dismissed (ie, "I'm not familiar with that diet") or their questions are ignored (ie, "Just feed a good-quality kibble or canned food"), this is not in the best interests of the patient. If

Table 1
American Pet Products Association National Pet Owner Survey responses when asked the "type of food used most often in 2010"

Product Position	Dog Owners (% of 544)			Cat Owners (% of 483)		
	Dry	Canned	Semimoist	Dry	Canned	Semimoist
Food fortified with nutrients	71	13	5	73	24	2
Food fortified with supplements	55	11	5	62	14	5
Food fortified with herbs/ botanicals	53	6	12	49	14	3
Food fortified with pre- or probiotics	62	14	—	61	22	4
Food labeled as "organic"	67	7	10	35	20	5
Food labeled as "natural"	56	23	3	62	27	6
Food labeled as "gourmet"	37	46	19	35	61	9
Food labeled as "premium"	82	20	9	76	27	3
Food – no special features	76	23	8	78	43	8
Human foods (cooked or raw)	9	4	10	8	12	7
Frozen food	33	—	17	50	75	25
Vegetarian food	43	29	—	75	75	25
Raw food	30	10	20	64	64	36

Percent may exceed 100 because owners are feeding more than one type of food.
Data from American Pet Products Association (APPA). National pet owner survey 2011–2012. Greenwich, CT: APPA; 2013.

a veterinarian does not provide advice with respect to alternative diets, then the pet owner turns to less-reliable sources for this information (eg, "Dr Google," pet chat forums, pet store employees). Thus, the goal of this article is to provide a practical approach to alternative diets for veterinarians in practice.

Dietary Options Available to Owners

It is a daunting task for any veterinarian to keep up to date with all of the commercial dry and canned options available to pet owners, let alone keeping up to date with all of the alternative dietary options as well. Once a small niche, products such as fresh, refrigerated, frozen, and dehydrated pet food products are gaining popularity, such that their sales figures are now appearing in annual retail reports and marketing data.[10] These alternative diets may or may not be adequate as the sole source of nutrition. The other upcoming group of products for pets adding more confusion to diet selection are known as toppers, mixers, appetizers, gravies, waters, and gels,[11] which are designed to be highly palatable and, for now, unlikely to be adequate as the sole nutrition.

There are tens, if not hundreds, of thousands of pet food products and any product could be modified within 6 months. There is *no way* a practitioner can keep up with the vast number of pet food products available on the market, so more likely than not, clients will be naming pet foods and feeding product combinations that are *unfamiliar* to veterinarians (consider this is the new norm). This does not relieve veterinarians of the responsibility of determining if the diet being fed to the patient is nutritionally adequate. Feeding a single commercially manufactured kibble or canned food makes determining nutritional adequacy of the total diet easier; however, the survey data indicate few clients are routinely feeding just one product. It will take joint effort on the part of the owner, the practitioner, and other members of the veterinary health care team to determine if the total diet is nutritionally adequate.

Our approach is based on the nutritional adequacy of these dietary options (ie, is the diet complete and balanced?). As shown in **Table 2**, we have developed 3 categories of nutritional adequacy under the following dietary options:

1. The product is adequate as the sole source of nutrition.
2. The product is inadequate as the sole source of nutrition but with instructions for the owner to nutritionally complete the diet (eg, add meat, oil, water, ± cooking).
3. The product is inadequate as the sole source of nutrition and no additional information is provided.

HOW TO ASSESS ALTERNATIVE DIETS

To aid veterinarians in assessing these unfamiliar products and combinations, a brief diet history (which the owner should ideally complete at home where they can see the exact name of all the products fed) should be completed before the appointment. Examples of such forms are readily available from the WSAVA Nutrition Toolkit (www. wsava.org/nutrition-toolkit). A useful diet history will name the manufacturer, product, life stage, form, amount fed, and number of meals (eg, Purina ONE SmartBlend Chicken and Brown Rice Entree canned, 1/2 can of a 368-g can, 3 times per day). Once this information becomes a part of the medical record (in a frequently seen portion that is easily checked at every visit similar to the vaccine history) then only updates are needed subsequently. If the owner purchases food from the veterinary clinic, records of food purchases are useful (eg, Royal Canin Veterinary Diet Gastrointestinal Low Fat canine canned, one 385-g can, divided into 2 meals per day). Pet owners are more likely to stick with the same or similar pet food products if they have their veterinarian's approval and continued assurance that their pet is being monitored for nutrition-related diseases using the AAHA[5] and WSAVA[6] Nutritional Assessment Guidelines (www.everypeteverytime.com/nutrition-assessment.html). One reason owners change pet food products or feed a combination of products may be they do not believe one product could be nutritionally complete for years. This notion of complete nutrition in one product contradicts the simple nutritional advice they were given for themselves (eg, eat a variety of foods).

It would be educational for the pet owner to learn how to determine the nutritional adequacy of all food and treat products fed to their pet. Initially to obtain this important information will require some upfront training of the owner on how to find, read, and interpret the nutritional adequacy statement on pet food labels. Once the owner has learned how to find and interpret the nutritional adequacy statement on pet foods, this skill will continue to be useful to them as they consider new pet food products coming onto the market at a regular pace. The AAHA Nutrition Reference Manual (www.everypeteverytime.com/docs/en-us/Pet_Nutrition_Ref_Manual.pdf) has an easy-to-understand explanation of Association of American Feed Control Officials (AAFCO) standards, pet food labeling, and nutritional adequacy statements available in a downloadable format. This type of client education and medical record entry is well within the skill set of most veterinary technicians.

North American Pet Food Regulations

Pet foods intended for sale in the United States will have an AAFCO statement of nutritional adequacy on the packaging, except if the product is clearly labeled as treat, snack, or supplement.[11] It is important to remember that AAFCO does not "police" the pet food industry. "AAFCO establishes the nutritional standards for complete

Table 2
Categorization of available dietary options based on nutritional adequacy

Available Dietary Options	Description	Nutritional Adequacy			Examples[a]
		Adequate as Sole Source of Nutrition	Inadequate as Sole Source of Nutrition with Instructions (Owner Required to Add Specific Ingredients per Instructions to Complete Adequacy)	Inadequate as Sole Source of Nutrition Without Instructions (Owner Required to Add Specific Ingredients but No Instructions Provided)	
1. Most commonly fed pet food products	Canned (ie, wet) or kibbled (ie, dry) food. Large-scale commercial production	Check nutritional adequacy statement.	—	Check nutritional adequacy statement.	"Canned or kibble diets," eg, Hill's Science Diet Adult dry, Friskies Classic Pate Chicken & Tuna Dinner canned
2. Homemade or home-prepared diets	Prepared at home by the owner after purchasing individual ingredients (eg, meats, grains, vegetables, vitamins, minerals).	Check credentials or guarantee of nutritional adequacy by originator of the recipe.	95% of available recipes cannot be used as sole source of nutrition.[42]		"Homemade diets," eg, www.Petdiets.com, www.BalanceIT.com, www.Homemadedogfood.com, www.Allrecipes.com
3. Premade "homemade" diets	Product is prepared commercially to resemble homemade diet. Preserved as shelf-stable or frozen.	Check credentials of originator or nutritional adequacy statement on the label.	—	Check credentials of originator or nutritional adequacy statement on the label.	"Re-invention of the TV dinner," eg, www.Raynenutrition.com, www.Freshpet.com, www.Freshwholefoodsfordog.com

4. Premade products	Premade blend of ingredients. Owner is required to make additions to the diet (eg, meat, oil, water) and ± cook the product.	No	Nutritional adequacy depends on the competency of the instructions provided and owner's ability to comply with instructions.	Inadequate if instructions are not correct or followed exactly by the owner.	"Re-invention of Hamburger Helper," eg, Balance IT Original Blends, Dr Harvey's Veg-to-Bowl
5. Mixers and toppers	Frozen, dehydrated, canned (usually game or novel) meat. Sometimes vegetables.	No	If product is used as part of a complete and balanced homemade diet recipe from a reputable originator.	If only product being fed to the pet. If the rest of the diet was invented by owner or recipe is not from a reputable source.	"Packaged meats/veggies," eg, Raw dehydrated medallions, frozen chubs, canned meat "au jus," self-stable cooked kangaroo, garden vegetable blends, canned pumpkin
6. Veterinary therapeutic diets	Canned or kibbled large-scale commercial production. Alternative is homemade diets.	Check nutritional adequacy statement, which often indicates product should be fed under the supervision of a veterinarian with appropriate monitoring, or check credentials of originator of recipe.	—	—	"Veterinary diets," eg, Hill's, Iams, Purina, Royal Canin, Rayne Clinical Nutrition, www.BalanceIT.com, www.Petdiets.com
Any combination(s) of the above (1–5)	Owner may choose any combination of homemade diet + premade products	If all products and recipes are complete and balanced, the final mix will most likely be adequate	—	Combining nutritionally inadequate products and recipes rarely (if ever) makes a complete and balanced diet by chance	"Eat a little bit of everything and it all comes out in the wash," eg, mixing canned and dry food, mixing homemade diet with canned food, adding human food to dry dog food

a The examples are for illustration purposes and do not by any means cover the entire breadth of examples available for each category.

and balanced pet foods, and *it is the pet food company's responsibility* to formulate their products according to the appropriate AAFCO standard."[12] It is the feed-control officials of each state that have the responsibility of *monitoring and regulating pet foods* (ie, ensuring all laws and rules set by the state with respect to pet food safety and manufacturing are abided by).[12] The *rare* exception would be pet foods that are manufactured within states that do not have regulations for manufacturing pet foods when these pet foods are not sold across state lines (eg, Alaska and Nevada).[13]

However, manufacturers of Canadian pet foods, intended for sale only in Canada, do not always take into account AAFCO's nutritional standards. Based on the authors' experience, it is not uncommon to encounter pet foods manufactured in Canada that lack a nutritional adequacy statement. The AAFCO Web site states, "Canada does not regulate pet food."[13] Although it is true that Canada has not officially adopted AAFCO's nutritional standards for complete and balanced pet foods, pet foods in Canada are *not* completely unregulated. For example, the Canadian Food Inspection Agency regulates importation of pet foods (containing animal products) and meat products.[14,15] Health Canada prohibits unsubstantiated health claims on pet foods and the Competition Bureau of Industry Canada has minimal labeling requirements for pre-packaged pet foods (ie, product name, net quantity, dealer's name and address).[15] False advertising and misleading information is also prohibited by the Competition Bureau. Thus, Canadian veterinarians should *only* recommend pet foods with AAFCO statements to ensure nutritional adequacy based on the more liberal nature of regulations for Canadian pet foods.

Determining Nutritional Adequacy of a Patient's Diet

There are 3 simple questions to ask when determining nutritional adequacy:

1. What type of nutritional adequacy statement is on the product?
2. Is the nutritional adequacy statement appropriate for this patient?
3. Has the specific product been recalled (typically recalls are by production lot or by brand)?

The AAFCO nutritional adequacy statement is the *most important* preliminary piece of information on the pet food label when assessing the diet for a particular patient. The statement will be 1 of only 3 options:

1. Nutritionally complete and balanced (or perfect, scientific, 100% nutritious) for a specific life stage (eg, adult maintenance, growth) or multiple life stages (eg, all life stages)
2. For intermittent or supplemental feeding only, or
3. Feed under the supervision or direction of a veterinarian.[16]

Nutritionally complete and balanced

Nutritionally complete and balanced (eg, perfect, scientific, 100% nutritious, total nutrition, balanced diet) diets are either formulations known to contain all required nutrients or shown to be nutritionally complete and balanced for dogs and cats of a specific life stage or life stages via feeding trials.[16] These diets can be fed to dogs or cats as the sole source of nutrition. Embedded in this complete and balanced statement will be the (1) species, (2) life stage, and (3) method of determining nutritional adequacy.[17]

Species For healthy pets, cat food should be fed to cats and dog food should be fed to dogs. When cat food is fed to dogs, it will likely provide excessive amounts of fat, calories, and possibly protein for a typical healthy adult dog. Dog food should be fed to dogs only, because the complete list of essential nutrients for cats would most likely be missing in a food formulated for dogs (eg, arginine, taurine, arachidonic acid).[17]

Some products on the market claim to have nutritional adequacy for both dogs and cats, which means the nutrient profile has to fit the species with more stringent requirements, which would be cats (so these are cat foods). The most relevant point here is that feline products would in all probability be excessive in calories for most adult neutered dogs.

Life stage There are 3 life stage claims possible: (1) gestation-lactation-growth, (2) adult or maintenance, and (3) all life stages.[17] A combination of life stages is also possible (eg, growth and maintenance).[17] The nutrient profile for gestation-lactation-growth is the most nutritionally demanding. Therefore, a food with an "all" life stages claims must meet the nutritional demands of gestation-lactation-growth of whichever species (dog or cat) it is intended (so these are puppy or kitten foods). The clinically relevant point here is that some of these all life-stage products (regardless of whether they are suitable for dog or cat) would potentially be excessive in calories for many sedentary, indoor, adult neutered dogs and cats. "All life stages" claims sound convenient to owners, but if these products have a higher caloric density and higher fat content to meet the needs of gestation-lactation-growth, then it is possible that these products will contribute to overweightness and obesity in sedentary, indoor, adult neutered dogs and cats. This has been the clinical impression of the authors at their respective institutions.

Method of determining nutritional adequacy There are only 2 methods for determining nutritional adequacy: (1) computer formulated based on nutrient requirements or (2) feeding trials using dogs or cats.[17] The preferred method of nutritional adequacy verification is the *feeding* method, where the food was fed to adult animals of the appropriate species as the sole source of nutrition for at least 6 months. AAFCO feeding trials for growth last 10 weeks, because nutritional deficiencies should develop more quickly during this stage because puppies and kittens have the strictest nutrient requirements. Gestation-lactation-growth (or all life stage) feeding trials follow the complete reproductive cycle and last a minimum of 26 weeks. AAFCO has feeding trial protocols that specify the length of the trial, number of dogs or cats, feeding procedures, and diagnostic tests needed to deem the feeding trial successful.[17] Feeding trials are the current gold standard, because feeding trials substantiate the bioavailability of the diet in addition to the nutritional adequacy. However, a product carrying a nutritional adequacy statement by either method is worthy of close monitoring as with any new dietary product.

AAFCO feeding trials require additional time and significant expense compared with computer-formulated diets. Unfortunately, in this age of marketing using negative statements, "no animal testing" claims in defense of computer-formulated diets is something the authors have encountered. Feeding 16 dogs or cats (8 control diet vs 8 test diet) as part of a 26-week feeding trial would not be considered invasive research by most standards.[17] The dogs and cats involved in feeding trials will also receive 2 physical examinations (by veterinarians), weekly body weight measurements, daily food intake measurements, and blood will be drawn at the end of the trial (eg, hemoglobin, albumin, taurine in cats). These routine measurements and tests should be completed annually in pet dogs and cats. Additionally, urine and feces may be collected for determining the metabolizable energy of the pet food,[17] which are also noninvasive procedures.

Action The most common mismatch is an owner feeding a high caloric density (high-fat) food to a middle-aged, inactive/obese-prone, neutered dog that already has a body condition score (BCS) greater than a 5/9 or to the middle-aged, indoor/sedentary, neutered cat with a BCS greater than 5/9. It would not take very long to help the owner determine such a product was inappropriate for their pet and to help them select a more appropriate adult maintenance product (with lower caloric density and fat) to maintain a healthier weight and body condition. Because of the enormous variation in the caloric densities and fat contents of all life stages products, both of these parameters should be assessed in addition to the AAFCO statement.

Intermittent or supplemental feeding only

For products with "intermittent or supplemental feeding only" claims, it is assumed or known to be nutritionally incomplete as the sole source of nutrition for an extended time period.[17] Over-the-counter products with this claim are not nutritionally adequate and if fed as the sole source of nutrition or even in combination with other pet foods carrying the same claim, are likely to cause a nutrition-related diseases within week to months, or possibly years depending on the problematic nutrients. The specific clinical sign that may appear first is dependent on the first limiting nutrient and magnitude of the variance from the recommended level (ie, toxicity vs deficiency); hence, one cannot predict the clinical signs of malnutrition without knowing the exact nutrient profile of the nutritionally inadequate product. The *exception* to this rule applies to veterinary therapeutic diets, as some of these products deliberately have an intermittent feeding claim regardless of nutritional adequacy.

Action Again, it would be well worth the time and effort needed to help the owner determine if such a product was inappropriate for their pet in the long term and to help the owner select a product with a complete and balanced nutritional adequacy statement.

Feed under the supervision or direction of a veterinarian

Products with a "feed under the supervision of a veterinarian" claim are reserved for the products used for specific medical conditions, for which direct veterinary supervision is required regardless of the diet being fed (Group 6, see **Table 2**).[17] Dietary examples include struvite dissolution, urolith prevention, chronic renal disease, liver disease with hepatic encephalopathy, weight loss, and so forth. It does not mean these diets contain nutrient excesses or deficiencies; in fact many of these therapeutic diets have passed AAFCO protocol feeding trials conducted within the company's research and development centers.

These products with a narrow margin of safety for certain essential nutrients carry very specific instructions about how to monitor the patient while consuming the diet. One of the best examples of such diets is Hill's Prescription Diet u/d Canine Non-Struvite Urinary Tract Health canned and dry diets.[18] The protein in the canned and dry diets are 2.9 g per100 kcal (13.3% on a dry matter basis [DMB]) and 2.5 g per 100 kcal (10.9% DMB), respectively. Thus, it is recommended in the product guide that patients on these diets are monitored for signs of protein depletion by using a fasting serum biochemistry panel and echocardiogram every 6 months (ie, under veterinary supervision).[18] The precautions *do not preclude* using these diets in *appropriately selected cases*. The nutrient profile in these diets meet National Research Council (NRC) minimal protein requirements for dogs (2.0 g/100 kcal or 8.0% DMB),[19] whereas AAFCO nutrient profiles use a larger margin of safety for adult dogs without nutrient-responsive disease (5.14 g/100 kcal or 18.0% DMB).[17] Per AAFCO recommendations, these diets are not nutritionally adequate for adult maintenance; however, these diets meet the minimal protein recommendations of the NRC.

Another example is Hill's Prescription Diets s/d Canine Dissolution canned,[18] which carries very specific instructions regarding the length of time this product can be fed ($\leq$6 months) and the product guide recommends the use of appropriate antibiotic therapy when a urinary tract infection is present. The protein level in this product falls below the protein requirements of adult dogs as determined by the NRC (2.0 g/100 kcal or 8.0% DMB)[19] so as to dissolve struvite stones and crystals (1.7 g/100 kcal or 7.9% DMB),[18] hence the time limit on feeding this diet.

Action The responsibility for closely monitoring nutrition-related clinical signs lies with the prescribing veterinarian. We recommend reading the product guide and/or contacting the manufacturer of the therapeutic diet for additional information on monitoring recommendations or clinical trials *before* recommending the product. That way the owner can be made aware of the essential need for monitoring when prescribing the therapeutic diet for a particular disease state.

Product recalls Once the nutritional adequacy statement has been checked on a particular product, it is unlikely to change unless recalled for a diet formulation error and then it should appear on the Food and Drug Administration (FDA) Pet Food Recall List (www.fda.gov/AnimalVeterinary/SafetyHealth/RecallsWithdrawals/default.htm). Naming a pet food brand or manufacturer you are familiar with does not preclude formulation errors. There were more than 30 recalls in 2013,[20] and some of the products were from familiar "major" pet food companies. Pet food product recalls are now very easy to check on the FDA Pet Food Recall List. Additionally, there are several other Web sites maintaining recall lists (eg, www.apsca.org, www.avma.org, www.animalhealthfoundation.net).

It is of the utmost importance to remind your clients that recalls are done to *protect* their pets (eg, nutrient deficiencies or excesses, bacterial contamination) and in some cases to *protect* the owner as well (eg, bacterial contamination). Avoid recommending foods that advertise negative claims, such as "no recalls ever," because yes recalls can be avoided altogether if a company is not responsibly testing pet food for problems. Product monitoring and recalls are part of the responsible manufacturing process.

Products without a nutritional adequacy statement AAFCO label regulations do not distinguish between alternative, commercial kibble, and commercial canned pet foods. Often the nutritional adequacy statement for these alternative products will be for "intermittent or supplemental feeding only," but some are complete and balanced as verified by the formulation method (see **Table 2**). One cannot assume nutritional inadequacy of a product simply because the diet is considered to be an alternative to dry kibble or canned pet foods.

Premade "homemade" diets Premade "homemade" diets are pet diets that resemble home-prepared diets from a pet owner's kitchen and provide the convenience of being commercially manufactured in ready-to-serve containers for owners to purchase. Some products from the premade homemade diet group (Group 3, see **Table 2**) carry a complete and balanced claim (eg, veterinary products from Rayne Clinical Nutrition at www.raynenutrition.com), whereas others that are similar in appearance have an intermittent or supplemental feeding only claim (eg, Fresh Whole Food for Dogs at www.freshwholefoodfordogs.com). The major difference between these 2 examples is the addition of specific vitamins and minerals, and adjusting the nutrient concentrations for the caloric density of the product, both of which require nutritional expertise to accomplish and is beyond the abilities of most individuals who prepare the diets in their homes and sell locally. This information may not be on the Web site or on promotional materials (because those items are not reviewed by state feed officials), but is required on the label of products sold in the United States if in a state that has adopted AAFCO guidelines.

Premade products Premade products (Group 4, see **Table 2**) are typically vegetable or novel carbohydrate blends that require the addition of ingredients like meat, oil, and water, and may or may not require cooking. These products may or may not contain essential vitamins and minerals. These premade products are not complete and balanced as a standalone diet; however, some provide specific mixing instructions to make the product complete and balanced provided the owner is compliant and understands the instructions. The products usually carry an intermittent or supplemental feeding claim. An AAFCO nutritional adequacy claim *cannot* be made for the final meal prepared at home by the owner. Dr Harvey's Veg-to-Bowl (www.drharveys.com), for example, provides instructions to make a "complete meal" implying the resulting meal will be nutritionally complete, but there is no nutritional guarantee stated.[21] This product's Web site claims the final meal prepared by the owner can be fed to puppies, adults, or overweight dogs, implying it is suitable for growth (ie, positive energy balance) and weight loss (ie, negative energy balance) at the same time; however, the product itself carries an intermittent or supplemental feeding claim.[21] Another concern is that the amount of protein and oil to be added to the premade product is left up to the discretion of the owner (eg, "Step 1. Add hot water to Veg-to-Bowl. Step 2. Let sit 8–10 minutes until cool. Step 3. Add protein of your choice. Step 4. Add oil. Step 5. Watch a Happy and Healthy Dog Eat!").[21]

Balance IT Blend products (secure.balanceit.com) (Group 4, see **Table 2**) infer nutritional adequacy because the products and instructions were designed by an American College of Veterinary Nutrition (ACVN at www.acvn.org/) board-certified veterinary nutritionist and detailed instructions are provided based on the weight of the pet being fed the product, but the product itself carries an intermittent or supplemental feeding claim.[22] In actuality, in both examples, the nutrient intake of the pet is not known completely unless veterinarians review the mixing instructions with the person who feeds the pet.

Mixers and toppers Mixers and toppers (Group 5, see **Table 2**), such as Wellness 95% Salmon Recipe canned (containing salmon, water sufficient for processing, natural flavors, cassia gum, and carrageenan), has an intermittent or supplemental feeding claim and under the feeding guidelines instructs the owner to use the product as a mixer or topper for dry kibble.[23] No proportions are offered to ensure the owner adds the correct amount of the canned meat product to the kibble to avoid unbalancing the nutrient profile of the complete and balanced kibble.[23] It is possible for the owner to overfeed this mixer or topper such that the nutrient intake by the pet is deficient in some micronutrients. The suggestion should be to limit the amount of mixers or toppers to less than 10% of the daily caloric intake (**Table 4**). Another example of a mixer or topper would be Wysong Beef AuJus canned (containing beef, water sufficient for processing, beef liver, animal plasma, and guar gum).[24]

Homemade or home-prepared diets The APPA National Pet Owners Survey reported 21% of dog owners and 15% of cat owners fed human foods or a homemade diet to their pets.[8] Homemade diets (Group 2, see **Table 2**) do not carry any nutritional adequacy statement; however, since the 2007 major pet food recall, the availability of homemade diet recipes has exploded. Recipes are readily available in popular press pet books, textbooks, chat rooms, blogs, and Web sites from the pet owner, neighbor, family, friends, breeders, veterinarians, and various types of nutritionists (eg, animal, human, and veterinary). Importantly, only veterinarians and animal nutritionists are likely to be held legally accountable for their recommendations based on their training.

There are 3 major areas of concern with homemade diets:

1. Is the nutrient profile appropriate?
2. Does the client make the recipe according to instructions?
3. Has the client deviated from the original recipe (ie, diet drift)?

Each of these areas of concerns have been reported to cause malnutrition in pets.[25–31]

Checking the nutritional adequacy of recipes is not a simple task and is most often beyond the skill set and time available to most practitioners. To correctly assess the nutrient profile of a homemade diet requires software, formulation skills, nutritional knowledge, and access to databases of available ingredients. Therefore, practitioners should be willing to:

- Assess the homemade diet recipe for 5 key nutrient sources and refer to a veterinary nutritionist if any nutrient source is missing (**Table 3**).[32]
- Offer nutritionally adequate recipes formulated by veterinary nutritionists.
- If a specific dietary formulation is necessary for medical reasons, help the client obtain advice from a veterinary nutritionist.

Boarded veterinary nutritionists (www.acvn.org/ and www.esvcn.com/), like other veterinary specialists, have advanced training and can be of particular assistance with homemade diets. Boarded veterinary nutritionists should be able to help balance most recipes if the owner insists on feeding particular ingredients. Practitioners can initially screen a recipe for nutritional adequacy by answering a short list of questions (see **Table 3**).[32] If the recipe fails or is questionable in any area, the practitioner should refer the client to a nutritionist if the client wishes to continue feeding that recipe. It is also important that, once the homemade diet has been documented as nutritionally sound, the recipe specifics are maintained in the medical record and reviewed on a regular basis with the owner to control for recipe deviations or diet drift over time (a common problem with homemade diets).

Determining product safety Although not directly a nutritional issue, it is also pertinent to ask, "Is this product safe to feed to the pet?" Not only does the health of the pet and owner hinge on this question, a veterinarian could be held legally accountable for either recommending or ignoring unsafe feeding practices. Raw meat and eggs, even if sold as "human-grade" or for "human consumption," can be contaminated with pathogenic bacteria (eg, *Salmonella, Escherichia coli, Clostridium, Campylobacter,* and *Listeria*).[33] It is important to note that freezing, freeze-drying, or high-pressure processing are not effective means of destroying these pathogens to guarantee safety.[31] Thus, animal proteins should be cooked to an internal temperature of 180°F (or 80° Celsius) for at least 10 minutes to ensure food safety.

Another safety concern pertains to feeding bones. The FDA has a handout in downloadable format that veterinarians can provide to owners who feed bones to their pets (at   www.fda.gov/downloads/ForConsumers/ConsumerUpdates/UCM209196.pdf). Among the many concerns with feeding bones to pets are the following[33,34]:

- Fractured teeth
- Mouth or jaw injuries

Table 3
Quick assessment of homemade diet recipes for veterinary practitioners

- Review each of the following aspects of the diet.
- If the response is *affirmative (YES)* for each section, the practitioner may with some assurance believe the diet will most likely meet the nutritional needs of most companion dogs and cats.
- If the response to any 1 of these 5 criteria is *negative (NO)* or *uncertain*, then the practitioner should not endorse the homemade recipe without confirmation from a qualified nutritionist.

Response		Dietary Sources
Yes	No	Protein (meat) source
		The final diet should contain 25%–30% cooked meat for dogs (1 part meat to 2 or 3 parts grain) and 35%–50% cooked meat for cats (1 part meat to 1 to 2 parts grain).
		The overall protein quality (amino acid profile) in a homemade food is good to excellent with animal (muscle or organ meat) protein. Liver or egg (25% of protein portion) can correct most potential amino acid deficiencies in homemade diets using vegetable protein sources.[a]
		In an ovo-lacto vegetarian diet for dogs, eggs are the best protein.[a]
		In a vegan diet for dogs, high-protein (eg, soy, pinto, or garbanzo) beans provide the next best, but incomplete, amino acid profile for dogs.[a]
Yes	No	Carbohydrate (grain) source
		A grain generally supplies little protein and mostly carbohydrate (as starch) for energy. The grain should be in greater quantity than the meat to keep the total protein less than 50%. Optimal grain-to-meat ratios should be at least 2:1 to 3:1 for dog foods and 1:1 to 2:1 for cat foods. Cooked corn, rice, wheat, potato, or barley are greater than 85% digested by both dogs and cats. If more fiber is need in the diet, the grain could be brown rice, sweet potato, or oatmeal.
Yes	No	Lipid (fat or oil) source
		A separate source of fat may or may not be present and the diet still be adequate. However, if a more calorie-dense diet is required (ie, more calories per volume), add fat to the diet to regain or maintain body weight and condition, and increase palatability. If the specified meat source is "lean" (eg, white or game meats), an additional animal, vegetable, or fish fat source may be needed. Changing the cut of meat (eg, sirloin to chuck) or fat content (eg, 10%–35%) in ground meat will also increase the fat content of the whole diet and provide essential fatty acids. All types of fat (animal [eg, butter, poultry skin, or meat trimmings], vegetable, or fish oils) can be used for added calories.
Yes	No	Calcium source
		Homemade diets require a specific calcium supplement and most often no additional phosphorous is need. Readily available calcium carbonate fed at 0.5 g/4.5-kg cat/d and at least 2.0 g/15-kg dog/d will most likely be appropriate for a diet with the previously mentioned meat and grain proportions.
Yes	No	Multivitamin and trace mineral source
		Supplements providing vitamins and minerals are not optional. These nutrient requirements cannot be met using "whole" foods, such as fruits and vegetables, because the pet simply cannot consume enough vegetable material to meet the stated Association of American Feed Control Officials recommendations. Therefore, synthetic supplements are required to ensure a complete diet.

[a] Vegetarian and vegan diets should not be fed to cats.
From Remillard RL, Crane SW. Making pet foods at home. In: Hand MS, Thatcher CD, Remillard RL, et al, editors. Small animal clinical nutrition. 5th edition. (KS): Mark Morris Institute; 2010. p. 207–23; with permission.

- Obstructions (eg, esophagus, trachea, stomach, small intestine, colon, rectum)
- Complications of obstructions (eg, sepsis, peritonitis)
- Constipation

HOW TO ASSESS PATIENTS ON ALTERNATIVE DIETS

Patients will be at risk for nutrition-related diseases if fed a nutritionally incomplete or improperly balanced diet long term (regardless of the manufacturer, how the product is positioned in the market place, or even if the product is familiar to the veterinarian). Based on the WSAVA[6] Nutritional Assessment Guidelines (www.everypeteverytime. com/nutrition-assessment.htm), nutritional assessment is considered the "5th Vital Assessment Group." The other 4 vital signs include temperature, pulse, respiration, and pain assessment. Making nutrition part of the vital assessment for each patient highlights the importance of proper nutrition for every single patient. If there are no nutritional risk factors (**Box 1**) present during the visit, then only the initial screening needs to be performed for that patient. However, if any nutritional risk factors are present (see **Box 1**), an extended nutritional evaluation must be performed. Additionally, *every patient consuming more than 10% of his or her total calories from alternative pet foods* should receive an extended nutritional evaluation, as illustrated in **Fig. 1**.

Box 1
Nutritional risk factors for patients

Patient History:

- Abnormal gastrointestinal function (eg, vomiting, nausea, diarrhea, increased frequency of defecation, flatulence, borborygymus, constipation)

- Preexisting medical conditions or disease states

- Receiving medications or dietary supplements

- *Consuming an unfamiliar or unknown to be nutritionally adequate diet* (see **Table 2**)

- *Consuming an unsafe (eg, raw animal proteins or bones) or a recalled diet*

- *Treats, snacks, human foods >10% of total caloric intake* (see **Table 4**)

- Inappropriate/inadequate housing/shelter

Physical Examination:

- Thin body condition (body condition score [BCS] <4 of 9)

- Overweight (BCS of 6–7 of 9) or obese body condition (BCS ≥8 of 9)

- Unintended or unexplained weight loss or weight gain

- Abnormal muscle condition score (ie, mild, moderate, or severe muscle wasting)

- Poor skin and coat quality

- Dental disease or abnormalities

- New medical conditions or disease states

Adapted from American Animal Hospital Association (AAHA) Nutritional Guidelines Taskforce. AAHA nutritional assessment guidelines for dogs and cats. J Am Anim Hosp Assoc 2010;46: 285–96; and The World Small Animal Veterinary Association (WSAVA) Nutritional Assessment Guidelines Task Force. WSAVA nutritional assessment guidelines. J Feline Med Surg 2011;13:516–25.

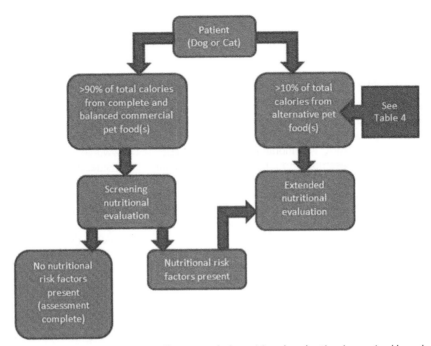

Fig. 1. Algorithm for determining if an extended nutritional evaluation is required based on the proportion of the diet the patient is consuming from complete and balanced commercial pet food(s) versus alternative pet food(s) based on AAHA[5] and WSAVA[6] Nutrition Assessment Guidelines. (*Adapted from* American Animal Hospital Association (AAHA) Nutritional Guidelines Taskforce. AAHA nutritional assessment guidelines for dogs and cats. J Am Anim Hosp Assoc 2010;46:285–96; and The World Small Animal Veterinary Association (WSAVA) Nutritional Assessment Guidelines Task Force. WSAVA nutritional assessment guidelines. J Feline Med Surg 2011;13:516–25.)

It is difficult to quickly assess what represents 10% of total calories for a patient. Ideally the number of calories consumed per day by the patient would be determined from a thorough dietary history. Then 10% of calories could be estimated and if the patient is consuming more than 10% of calories from alternative pet food(s), then an extended evaluation should be performed. However, not every owner can provide a thorough dietary history. This could be because multiple people are responsible for feeding the pet or the pet's diet may be so varied from day to day that calculating the number of calories consumed daily becomes a challenge. Under these circumstances, we recommend using **Table 4** to help determine what 10% of the total amount of food being consumed daily is (either in wt-oz or grams), based on a pet consuming approximately 2% of their body weight in food daily. For example, a 50-lb (22.7-kg) dog would consume approximately 16 wt-oz (455 g) of food per day. Thus, 10% of the total daily food intake would be 1.6 wt-oz (45 g). If the patient is consuming more than 1.6 wt-oz (45 g) of an unknown product or a product with an intermittent or supplemental feeding claim, then an extended nutritional evaluation should be performed (see **Fig. 1**).

Table 4 is also useful for determining an appropriate number of treats to allow a patient to consume daily in addition to a complete and balanced pet food. Because treats are most often nutritionally incomplete, they are intended for intermittent or

Table 4
Determine if a patient is consuming more than 10% of total daily calories from nutritionally incomplete or unbalanced products based on body weight

Body Weight[a]	Total Daily Intake[b]	10% of Total Daily Calories			Approximate Daily Energy Requirements[c]	Total Daily Intake[b]	Body Weight[a]
lb	Wt-oz of Food	kcal	Wt-oz of Food	Grams of Food	kcal/d	Grams of Food	kg
5	2	16	0.2	5	155	45	2.3
10	3	26	0.3	9	261	91	4.5
15	5	35	0.5	14	354	136	6.8
20	6	44	0.6	18	440	182	9.1
25	8	52	0.8	23	520	227	11.4
30	10	60	1.0	27	596	273	13.6
35	11	67	1.1	32	669	318	15.9
40	13	74	1.3	36	740	364	18.2
45	14	81	1.4	41	808	409	20.5
50	16	87	1.6	45	874	455	22.7
60	19	100	1.9	55	1002	545	27.3
70	22	113	2.2	64	1125	636	31.8
80	26	124	2.6	73	1244	727	36.4
90	29	136	2.9	82	1359	818	40.9
100	32	147	3.2	91	1470	909	45.5
110	35	158	3.5	100	1579	1000	50.0
120	38	169	3.8	109	1686	1091	54.5
130	42	179	4.2	118	1790	1182	59.1
140	45	189	4.5	127	1893	1273	63.6
150	48	199	4.8	136	1993	1364	68.2

[a] Use current body weight for pets with ideal/underweight body condition scores and ideal body weight for pets with overweight/obese body condition scores.
[b] Estimated as approximately 2% of the patient's body weight.
[c] Using a factor of 1.2 times resting energy requirements (maintenance factor for neutered adult cats or inactive/obese-prone dogs).

supplemental feeding only and should make up less than 10% of daily intake to avoid unbalancing the nutrient profile of a pet's complete and balanced diet. Thus, the same 50-lb (22.7 kg) dog consuming approximately 16 wt-oz (455 g) of food per day, should receive less than 1.6 wt-oz (45 g) of treats per day.

Body Weight Trends, Body Condition Scores, and Muscle Condition Scores

Patient body weights are useful when looking at trends in body weight over time and help identify when unintentional weight gain or loss has occurred. However, the best assessment of whether or not a patient's body weight is ideal is to assess the patient's BCS as objectively as possible by referencing the WSAVA BCS charts for dogs and cats available at www.wsava.org/nutrition-toolkit. An ideal BCS is a 4 to 5 of 9 for dogs and cats.

Because BCS specifically assesses body fat, a muscle condition score (MCS) should always accompany a BCS. The MCS is determined by palpating muscle mass over boney prominences (eg, temporal bones, scapulae, spinous processes, ilial wings) and ranges from normal muscle condition to mild, moderate, or severe muscle wasting on the WSAVA MCS chart available at www.wsava.org/nutrition-toolkit. Muscle wasting tends to first become palpable along the epaxial muscles when the spinous processes become more pronounced and then tends to vary in other locations based on the patient.[6]

Any patient with unintentional weight changes and/or an abnormal BCS and MCS requires further dietary and medical investigation.

Feces

Increased frequency of defecation, soft stools, or diarrhea (small bowel vs large bowel), constipation (ie, <1 bowel movement in 24 hours), and flatulence are all important patient factors when it comes to assessing an animal consuming an alternative diet. Owners who feed raw-food diets (high in protein) often claim pets produce smaller and fewer stools. However, a dog or cat that defecates only once every 2 days has mild-moderate constipation, especially if the stools are hard, dry, and expelled as individual pellets. Normal feces should be firm, but not hard and have a segmented appearance.[35] The diet should be evaluated carefully in addition to medical reasons for abnormal feces.

Skin and Coat

Veterinarians should examine the skin and coat carefully in patients consuming alternative diets to assess for long-term (>3 months) dietary deficiencies or imbalances. Particular attention should be paid to patients with (1) dry or brittle hair coats; (2) hair coats that are sparse or easily plucked; (3) slow regrowth following clipping; (4) scaling, erythema, or crusting; (5) poor or delayed wound healing; and (6) changes in hair coat color.[6,36]

Baseline diagnostics, including a complete blood count, biochemistry panel, urinalysis, and thyroid assessment, should be performed to rule out systemic or metabolic causes of skin and coat abnormalities. Microscopic evaluation of plucked hairs (trichography) and examination of skin biopsies (dermatohistopathology) are the most useful when combined with dietary history for diagnosing nutrient-responsive dermatoses.[36] It is important to keep in mind that patients with higher nutrient requirements are more likely to present with nutrient-responsive dermatoses.[36] For example, dogs and cats that are growing, pregnant or lactating, or recovering from illness are more likely to be at risk. If any of the nutrient concerns listed in the following paragraph are suspected based on dietary history and assessment of the skin and coat, the best approach is to transition the patient to a known complete and balanced diet that has undergone an AAFCO feeding trial to substantiate nutrient bioavailability. If that is not possible, then a veterinary nutritionist should be consulted for advice on balancing the alternative diet.

Protein-energy malnutrition can lead to (1) sparse hair coat or alopecia with hairs that are easily plucked, (2) abnormal keratinization, (3) coat color changes, and (4) impaired wound healing or ulcerations.[36] Patients with these clinical signs may have been consuming an alternative diet that provided dietary protein and energy at levels lower than required. Additionally, the protein source in the alternative diet may be poorly digestible (ie, dry matter digestibility <60%), poorly bioavailable (eg, high fiber content in high-protein beans), or may not have supplied all essential amino acids (eg, exclusively vegetable proteins being fed to cats).

For example, deficiency of the amino acids phenylalanine and tyrosine can result in lower melanin production, which results in hair coat color changes (eg, black to reddish brown).[36] Recall phenylalanine (an essential amino acid) can be converted to tyrosine, so tyrosine is not normally considered essential. However, under circumstances with higher essential amino acid requirements (eg, growth, gestation, lactation, illness) we may consider tyrosine conditionally essential if coat color changes are noted.

Essential fatty acid deficiency can manifest as (1) dull, dry hair coat; (2) scaling and erythema; (3) alopecia; (4) poor hair growth or regrowth; and (5) interdigital exudation.[36] Because the skin is the largest organ, it is prime target for essential fatty acid deficiency.[37] Additionally, linoleic fatty acid (18:2, ω-6) is important for maintaining the transepidermal moisture barrier.[37] Patients can develop essential fatty acid deficiency from consuming an alternative diet that lacks an appropriate fat source. Both cats and dogs have a nutrient requirement for omega-6 (ω-6) and omega-3 (ω-3) fatty acids.[37]

The skin is also affected by micronutrient deficiencies, such as zinc, copper, vitamin A, vitamin E, and/or B vitamins (eg, biotin and riboflavin).[36] It can be difficult or expensive to test for micronutrient deficiencies, so if the diet is unbalanced the best approach is to transition the patient to a known complete and balanced diet that has undergone an AAFCO feeding trial and monitor the patient over the next 6 months.

Eyes and Vision

Patients consuming unbalanced alternative diets long term that are deficient in retinol (ie, preformed vitamin A required by cats) or beta-carotene (ie, pro–vitamin A that can be converted to retinol by dogs and not cats) are at risk of vitamin A deficiency.[38] Patients with adequate stores of vitamin A (mainly in the liver) from previously eating a diet with adequate vitamin A will mobilize these stores while consuming a deficient diet. If a vitamin A–deficient diet is consumed long term (ie, 3–6 months, or longer, depending on the patient's prior stores and just how deficient the diet is), the patient's stores will become depleted. Vitamin A deficiency can result in ocular changes, such as night blindness (nyctalopia) and severe conjunctival dryness (xerophthalmia).[38] If an owner mentions any changes in the patient's visual abilities in dim lighting or at night (eg, walking into objects or difficulty walking at night), a complete visual examination should be performed. Vitamin A can be measured in the patient's serum or by using a liver biopsy sample. Vitamin A (eg, retinol and beta-carotene) also can be measured in the diet; however, these tests tend to be expensive and may have long turnaround times. The better approach is to transition the patient to a known complete and balanced diet that has undergone an AAFCO feeding trial. Also, ensure that owners do not go overboard supplementing vitamin A if you suspect deficiency, as vitamin A toxicity would not be in the best interests of the patient either.

Skeleton

One of the major concerns with unbalanced alternative diets is the lack of dietary calcium combined with high dietary phosphorus (typically coming from the high meat content of these alternative diets).[32] This results in an inverse calcium:phosphorus ratio. In general, calcium levels in the diet should be slightly higher than phosphorus levels, with an ideal ratio range of 1.1:1.0 to 2.0:1.0 (ie, 1.1 to 2.0 parts calcium for every 1.0 part phosphorus).[17] An inverse calcium-to-phosphorus ratio can result in the development of nutritional secondary hyperparathyroidism.[38] Patients attempt to maintain calcium homeostasis at all costs. This occurs primarily via the effects of parathyroid hormone (PTH) on bone resorption, resulting in decreased bone mineral density. Bone pain from microfractures or complete fractures is not uncommon with nutritional secondary hyperparathyroidism. Thus, sequential radiographs to assess bone density over time or to assess fracture healing become important while monitoring patients with decreased bone mineral density. Additionally, serum ionized calcium, 25-OH-D$_3$, and PTH should be monitored in these patients.

Laboratory Data

There is a tendency for owners to believe the diet fed to their pet is adequate if all of the routine blood parameters measured by the practitioner are within normal limits. This is not the case, as very few nutritional deficiencies or toxicities can be found on a routine complete blood count, serum biochemistry profile, or urinalysis. Baseline blood work can be useful from the standpoint of evaluating the patient's nutritional status grossly.[32] For example, red blood cells and hemoglobin can be assessed for iron-deficiency anemia or macrocytic anemia (ie, vitamin B12 or folate deficiencies). Blood albumin can act as an indicator of possible protein malnutrition. However, both albumin and red blood cell parameters require weeks to months of abnormal nutrient intakes before resulting in an abnormal test value. Additional diagnostics, such as vitamin B12, folate, ionized calcium, 25-OH-D$_3$, PTH, and iron studies, can be useful when clinical signs suggest abnormalities. However, assessing every micronutrient or hormone will not be cost or time effective for the veterinarian or patient. Again, the best approach is to transition the patient to a complete and balanced diet with continued monitoring and reassessment.

SUMMARY

A disparity in veterinary pet nutrition has been under way for some time, but has now become all too apparent. At a time when clients are motivated by a wide variety of reasons to consider alternative dietary products for their pets, veterinarians are less than adequately versed in pet nutrition and alternative dietary options. Increasing the pressure on this disparity are the dramatic advances in the understanding nutrition plays in health and disease. Key nutritional factors (ie, essential nutrients and bioactive food components) have been documented as potential modulators of health and disease.[39–41] Through nutrigenomics research, we are beginning to understand the ways in which food components affect gene expression directly and indirectly and, hence, modulate health and disease. Clients have already begun requesting such information for their dog and cat companions in this regard. To remain competitive, practitioners must consider raising their level of nutritional competency or incorporating the specialty of nutrition, through consultants if need be, into their practice to meet this growing client demand.

REFERENCES

1. Axelsson E, Ratnakumar A, Arendt ML, et al. The genomic signature of dog domestication reveals adaptation to a starch-rich diet. Nature 2013;495:360–4.
2. Crane SW, Cowell CS, Stout NP, et al. Commercial pet foods. In: Hand MS, Thatcher CD, Remillard RL, et al, editors. Small animal clinical nutrition. 5th edition. Topeka (KS): Mark Morris Institute; 2010. p. 157–90.
3. Case LP, Daristotle L, Hayek MG, et al. History and regulation of pet foods. In: Case LP, Daristotle L, Hayek MG, et al, editors. Canine and feline nutrition. 3rd edition. St. Louis (MO): Mosby; 2011. p. 121–9.
4. Laflamme DP, Abood SK, Fascetti AJ, et al. Pet feeding practices of dog and cat owners in the United States and Australia. J Am Vet Med Assoc 2008;232(5):687–94.
5. American Animal Hospital Association (AAHA) Nutritional Guidelines Taskforce. AAHA nutritional assessment guidelines for dogs and cats. J Am Anim Hosp Assoc 2010;46:285–96.

6. The World Small Animal Veterinary Association (WSAVA) Nutritional Assessment Guidelines Task Force. WSAVA nutritional assessment guidelines. J Feline Med Surg 2011;13:516–25.

7. Definition of "conventional." Available at: www.google.ca. Accessed October 27, 2013.

8. American Pet Products Association (APPA). National pet owner survey 2011-2012. Greenwich (CT): APPA; Canine p. 84; Feline p. 188.

9. Definition of "alternative." Available at: www.google.ca. Accessed October 27, 2013.

10. Taylor J. Market trends: pet food enhancers. In: Pet food industry. 2013. Available at: www.petfoodindustry-digital.com/201310/201310/15/0#&pageSet=15. Accessed October 27, 2013.

11. Association of American Feed Control Officials (AAFCO) website. Labeling and labeling requirements. Available at: petfood.aafco.org/LabelingLabelingRequirements.aspx#labeling. Accessed October 29, 2013.

12. Association of American Feed Control Officials (AAFCO). The business of pet food. Available at: www.petfood.aafco.org/. Accessed October 26, 2013.

13. Association of American Feed Control Officials (AAFCO). State feed program information. Available at: www.petfood.aafco.org/StateFeedProgramInformation.aspx. Accessed October 26, 2013.

14. Canadian Food Inspection Agency (CFIA). Pet food. Available at: www.inspection.gc.ca/animals/feeds/pet-food/eng/1299870750016/1320602183408. Accessed February 3, 2014.

15. Competition Bureau of Industry Canada. Guide for the labelling and advertising of pet foods. Available at: www.competitionbureau.gc.ca/eic/site/cb-bc.nsf/eng/01229.html#s1. Accessed February 3, 2014.

16. Association of American Feed Control Officials (AAFCO). Calorie content. Available at: www.petfood.aafco.org/CalorieContent.aspx. Accessed October 29, 2013.

17. Association of American Feed Control Officials (AAFCO). Model bill and regulations. In: AAFCO, editor. 2013 official publication. West Lafayette (IN): AAFCO; 2013. p. 90–205.

18. Hill's Pet Nutrition Canada, Inc. Key to clinical nutrition (product guide). 2011.

19. National Research Council (NRC). Nutrient requirements and dietary nutrient concentrations. In: NRC, editor. NRC nutrient requirements for dogs and cats. Washington DC (WA): The National Academies Press; 2006. p. 354–70.

20. Food and Drug Administration (FDA). Animal & veterinary recalls & withdrawals. Available at: www.fda.gov/animalVeterinary/safetyhealth/recallswithdrawals/default.htm. Accessed October 29, 2013.

21. Dr. Harvey's website. Veg-to-Bowl. Available at: www.drharveys.com/products/show/13-veg-to-bowl. Accessed October 27, 2013.

22. DVM Consulting, Inc. Balance IT original blends—oats for adult dogs. Available at: secure.balanceit.com/marketplace2.2/details.php?i=18&cc=. Accessed October 27, 2013.

23. Wellpet, LLC. Wellness 95% salmon recipe. Available at: www.wellnesspetfood.com/product-details.aspx?pet=dog&;pid=49. Accessed October 27, 2013.

24. Wysong. Wysong AuJus Diets. Available at: www.wysong.net/products/aujus-natural-healthy-dog-cat-ferret-food.php. Accessed January 16, 2014.

25. Streiff EL, Zwischenberger B, Butterwick RF, et al. A comparison of the nutritional adequacy of home-prepared and commercial diets for dogs. J Nutr 2002;132:1698S–700S.

26. Donoghue S, Kronfeld DS. Home-made diets. In: Wills JM, Simpson KW, editors. The Waltham book of clinical nutrition of dogs and cats. London: Pergamon; 1994. p. 445.

27. Roudebush P, Cowell CS. Results of a hypoallergenic diet survey of veterinarians in North America with a nutritional evaluation of homemade diet prescriptions. Vet Dermatol 1992;3:23–8.
28. Niza MM, Vilela CL, Ferreria LM. Feline pansteatitis revisited: hazards of unbalanced home-made diets. J Feline Med Surg 2003;5:271–7.
29. Polizpoulou ZS, Kazakos G, Patsikas MN, et al. Hypervitaminosis A in the cat: a case report and review of the literature. J Feline Med Surg 2005;7:363–8.
30. de Fornel-Thibaud P, Blanchard G, Escoffier-Chateau L, et al. Unusual case of osteopenia associated with nutritional calcium and vitamin D deficiency in an adult dog. J Am Anim Hosp Assoc 2007;43:52–60.
31. Gray CM, Sellon RK, Freeman LM. Nutritional adequacy of two vegan diets for cats. J Am Vet Med Assoc 2004;225(11):1670–5.
32. Remillard RL, Crane SW. Making pet foods at home. In: Hand MS, Thatcher CD, Remillard RL, et al, editors. Small animal clinical nutrition. 5th edition. Topeka (KS): Mark Morris Institute; 2010. p. 207–23.
33. Freeman LM, Chandler ML, Hamper BA, et al. Current knowledge about the risks and benefits of raw-meat based diets for dogs and cats. J Am Vet Med Assoc 2013;243(11):1549–68.
34. Food and Drug Administration. No bones about it: bones are unsafe for your dog. Available at: www.fda.gov/forconsumers/consumerupdates/ucm208365.htm. Accessed October 27, 2013.
35. Laflamme DP, Xu H, Cupp CJ, et al. Evaluation of canned therapeutic diets for the management of cats with naturally occurring chronic diarrhea. J Feline Med Surg 2012;14(10):669–77.
36. Roudebush P, Schoenher WD. Skin and hair disorders. In: Hand MS, Thatcher CD, Remillard RL, et al, editors. Small animal clinical nutrition. 5th edition. Topeka (KS): Mark Morris Institute; 2010. p. 637–65.
37. National Research Council. Fat and fatty acids. In: Nutrient requirements of dogs and cats. Washington DC (WA): National Academies Press; 2006. p. 81–110.
38. Wedekind KJ, Yu S, Kats L, et al. Micronutrients: minerals and vitamins. In: Hand MS, Thatcher CD, Remillard RL, et al, editors. Small animal clinical nutrition. 5th edition. Topeka (KS): Mark Morris Institute; 2010. p. 107–48.
39. Dove RS. Nutritional therapy in the treatment of heart disease in dogs. Altern Med Rev 2001;6:S38–45.
40. Deboer DJ. Canine atopic dermatitis: new targets, new therapies. J Nutr 2004; 134(8):2056S–61S.
41. Watson TD. Diet and skin disease in dogs. J Nutr 1998;128(12):2783S–9S.
42. Stockman J, Fascetti AJ, Kass PH, et al. Evaluation of recipes of home-prepared maintenance diets for dogs. J Am Vet Med Assoc 2013;242(11):1500–5.

Myths and Misperceptions About Ingredients Used in Commercial Pet Foods

Dottie Laflamme, DVM, PhD[a],*, Oscar Izquierdo, PhD[b],
Laura Eirmann, DVM[c], Stephen Binder, PhD[b]

KEYWORDS

• By-products • Corn • Soy • Wheat • Grains • Carbohydrates • Preservatives

KEY POINTS

- Ingredients used in pet food can be cause for concern among pet owners and veterinarians, in part, due to lack of knowledge about these ingredients.
- Ingredients used in pet food are selected primarily for their nutrient content, as well as their impact on palatability, digestibility, and consumer preferences.
- The finished product quality depends on selection of ingredients that provide the desired features, as well as the appropriateness of the processing and cooking processes.
- If veterinarians have questions about the quality of a food, they should contact the manufacturer and inquire about the nutrient profile and the digestibility of the product, which are good markers of the quality of the food.
- Veterinarians also should consider the history of the company, their pattern of investment into research, and their safety record when considering whether or not to recommend a product.

Ingredients used in pet food can be cause for concern among both pet owners and veterinarians, in part, due to lack of knowledge about these ingredients. Pet owners may not understand why "chemicals" are included in the food, when, in fact, those chemicals are actually essential vitamins or minerals. They may not be aware that "meat by-products" include most of the organs and other highly nutritious parts of the animal. Some of the concern is triggered by information and misinformation widely available through various sources including the Internet, popular publications, other pet owners, and even veterinarians. This article provides the facts regarding several commonly expressed concerns or myths regarding ingredients used in commercial pet foods beginning with definitions of some frequently misunderstood terms (**Box 1**).

[a] Nestlé Purina Research, Checkerboard Square, St. Louis, MO 63164, USA; [b] Product Technology Center, Nestlé Purina PetCare Company, Checkerboard Square, St Louis, MO 63164, USA; [c] Nestlé Purina PetCare Company, 54 Finch Road, Ringwood, NJ 07456, USA
* Corresponding author. Nestlé Purina PetCare Research, 473 Grandma's Place, Floyd, VA 24091.
E-mail address: Dorothy.laflamme@rd.nestle.com

Vet Clin Small Anim 44 (2014) 689–698
http://dx.doi.org/10.1016/j.cvsm.2014.03.002 **vetsmall.theclinics.com**

Box 1
Explanation of commonly used ingredient terms

AAFCO: The Association of American Feed Control Officials (http://www.aafco.org) is a voluntary membership association of local, state, and federal agencies charged by law to regulate the sale and distribution of animal feeds and animal drug remedies. Among their functions, they establish guidelines for pet foods in terms of nutritional guidelines and testing required to substantiate nutritional claims, and they define acceptable ingredients for use in animal feeds. Enforcement of these guidelines is done on a state by state level.

Animal or poultry digest: a highly palatable protein source that is made by chemical or enzymatic hydrolysis (digestion) of meat or poultry meat or by-products.

Beef tallow: fat derived from cattle.

BHA: butylated hydroxyanisole, an antioxidant used to protect dietary fats from becoming rancid.

Brewer rice: broken or small grains of white rice, they have the same nutritional value as intact white rice.

Corn gluten meal: a concentrated protein source derived from corn after removal of most of the starch, fiber, and oils. Although highly digestible, it requires a complementary source of lysine for optimum protein quality.

Flour: ingredient made from finely ground grains, which may or may not include the whole grain.

"Human grade": this term has no legal definition but implies that a food is suitable for human consumption. When one or more human edible ingredients are mixed with one or more nonhuman edible ingredients, the edible ingredients become nonhuman edible. According to AAFCO (http://petfood.aafco.org/LabelingLabelingRequirements.aspx), "human grade" claims should only be made if all ingredients, processing, and handling are such that the finished product is suitable for consumption by humans. If the finished product is not suitable for human consumption, then any claims related to "human grade" are considered misleading.

Meat by-products: a protein source consisting of organ meats, scrap meat, bone, blood, and fatty tissue from mammals, such as cattle or hogs. By-products do not include hair/hide, horns, hoofs or teeth, or intestinal contents.

Meat by-product meal: a concentrated protein source made by rendering[a] and drying meat by-products.

Menadione sodium bisulfite complex: provides a stable dietary source of Vitamin K.

Mixed tocopherols: natural source of Vitamin E and related compounds, used as an antioxidant to protect dietary fats from becoming rancid.

Natural: as defined by AAFCO, any feed or ingredient derived solely from plant, animal, or mineral sources can be labeled as natural. Any item synthesized chemically cannot be considered natural.

Organic: a food or ingredient that has been produced and handled in compliance with the requirements of the USDA National Organic Program. For example, organic grains are grown without the use of synthetic fertilizers and do not use genetic engineering. For more information, the reader is referred to the USDA website: http://www.ams.usda.gov/AMSv1.0/nop

Poultry by-products: a protein source consisting of the cleaned parts of slaughtered poultry to include the organs, heads, and feet. Poultry predominantly includes chickens and turkeys, but may include other birds raised for food.

Poultry by-product meal: a concentrated protein source made by rendering[a] and drying poultry by-products.

Soybean meal: a protein source derived from soybeans after removal of most of the starch, fiber, and oils. Although highly digestible, it requires a complementary source of methionine for optimum protein quality.

TBHQ: tertiary butyl hydroquinone, an antioxidant used to protect dietary fats from becoming rancid.

Wheat gluten: a concentrated protein source derived from wheat after removal of most of the starch, fiber, and oils. Used not only as a protein source but also for structural benefits, it is often added to baked goods (eg, breads and cakes) and other processed foods.

Whole grain: any grain that is included in its entirety, including the bran, germ, and endosperm. Ground, cracked, rolled, or otherwise processed whole grains may be called "whole grain" or "ground whole grains".

[a] See text for explanation of rendering.

GRAINS IN PET FOODS

Concerns about grains in pet foods seem to center on 3 points: (1) they are often called "fillers" or are said to have little nutritional value; (2) there are questions about the quality of grains used in pet food; and (3) they are reported to cause allergies.

Grains used in food include the true grains, derived from agricultural grasses, such as wheat, corn, rice, barley, rye, and oats, as well as the pseudograins such as quinoa, sorghum, millet, and others. The grain seed or kernel consists of the outer bran layer, endosperm, and germ. Whole grains, whether they are intact, cracked, rolled, or extruded contain the entire kernel. They are used in human and pet food for the nutritional value that they bring. Whole grains are not only a rich source of carbohydrates, which is the primary contribution, but also contain essential fatty acids, protein and essential amino acids, dietary fiber, and vitamins. Whole corn, for example, contains approximately 75% starch and other digestible carbohydrates, 6% to 10% protein, 4% to 5% fat, and 7% total dietary fiber.[1] Refining or processing grains can generate several coproducts that may concentrate on certain nutrients, such as protein, fiber, starch, or oils, and as processed and cooked such as in the making of pet foods, the carbohydrates, protein, and fat in grains are typically highly digestible.[2–6] Although there is no legal definition of "fillers", because the term is usually used to refer to feed ingredients with little or no nutritional value, grains should not be considered "fillers".

The United States Department of Agriculture (USDA) determines the quality criteria for whole grains. Administered by the USDA's Grain Inspection, Packers and Stockyards Administration (GIPSA; http://www.gipsa.usda.gov/fgismain.html), the Official US Standards for Grain provide criteria for determining the kind, class, and condition and quality of grains and oilseeds. Grains such as corn and wheat are graded according to a 5-point grading system, with Grades 1 and 2 being the higher quality corn. Grades 3 to 5 contain more moisture and can include more damaged kernels, which would make these grades more susceptible to mold or damage during storage. Grades 1 and 2, corn and wheat, are the predominant grades used in pet foods and in most processed foods for human consumption.

USDA standards define quality and set grade limits. Makers of high-quality pet foods, however, often use commercial specifications that are even more rigorous than the US Grain Standards when testing for evidence of damage or contamination, as well as nutritional standards. Although the details are proprietary and can vary among companies, sampling, grading, and testing occur even before the grains are unloaded at the facilities, and quality control measures continue throughout the storage, handling, and manufacturing processes, based on the company's standards.

Allergies and Grains

Food allergies or sensitivities are abnormal reactions to a normal food or ingredient. Although the true incidence of food allergies is unknown, they are considered to be uncommon, accounting for 1% of skin disease or less than 10% of allergic skin disease in dogs.[7] Food sensitivities can manifest with gastrointestinal signs, dermatologic signs, or both. The vast majority of allergens are proteins or glycoproteins. Because allergies are abnormal or inappropriate reactions of the immune system against a normal protein, they can form to any protein or protein-containing food or ingredient. The most commonly identified food allergens in dogs and cats are listed in **Table 1**.[7] Generally, the list reflects commonly fed ingredients.

Grains do contain protein, so allergies to grains can occur. Wheat, a commonly fed grain, is on the list of frequently identified allergens, accounting for 15% of the identified cases of food hypersensitivity in dogs and (in combination with barley) in about 5% in cats. Reactions to other grains and carbohydrate sources, such as rice, corn, and potato have been reported, but appear to be much less common. But because grains are very commonly fed and allergies to these are relatively uncommon, that is, less than 1.5% of pet allergies (based on the numbers cited earlier), there appears to be nothing inherently hyperallergenic in grains.

Celiac disease in humans is a heritable autoimmune disease associated with hypersensitivity to gluten proteins in wheat and related grains. Many celiac patients will also have an adverse reaction to barley and rye, as these grains are closely related. Corn gluten and rice gluten, on the other hand, are quite different from wheat gluten and can be consumed by most celiac patients without concern. A similar, heritable celiac-like disease has been observed in a small number of dogs, including some Irish Setters.[8] However, as previously noted, allergies to wheat and other grains are not common in dogs or cats.[7]

Carbohydrates in Pet Foods

Another commonly voiced concern about grains is that the carbohydrates they provide are not needed by dogs or, especially, cats. Some pet owners perceive that carbohydrates from grains and other sources are not digestible by dogs or cats. However, some pet owners will seek out foods with low or no grains, assuming this equates to low or no carbohydrate. In this section, the authors address the nutritional requirement, digestion, and metabolic use of dietary carbohydrates in cats and dogs and also discuss other nongrain sources of dietary carbohydrates used in pet foods.

Table 1	
Most commonly identified food allergens among dogs and cats with food hypersensitivities	
Dogs (N = 198)	**Cats (N = 89)**
Beef (36%)[a]	Beef (20%)
Dairy (28%)	Dairy (14.6%)
Wheat (15%)	Fish (13%)
Egg (10%)	Lamb (6.7%)
Chicken (9.6%)	Poultry (4.5%)
Lamb/mutton (6.6%)	Barley/wheat (4.5%)
Soy (6%)	

[a] Percentage refers to the percentage of total reported cases that were sensitive to the ingredient. Some patients were sensitive to more than one ingredient.

From Verlinden A, Hesta M, Millet S, et al. Food allergy in dogs and cats: a review. Crit Rev Food Sci Nutr 2006;46:268; with permission.

There is no evidence that adult, nonreproducing cats or dogs have a dietary requirement for carbohydrates, but this is true for most mammalian species, including humans.[9,10] Like other mammals, cats and dogs have a metabolic need for carbohydrates in the form of glucose, which is required by the brain and nervous tissues, red blood cells, renal medulla, and testes; the mammary gland during lactation; and the pregnant uterus.[11] When dietary carbohydrates are not provided, de novo gluconeogenesis, primarily from amino acids but also from the glycerol backbone of triglycerides, provides the required glucose. Because the physiologic requirement for carbohydrates can be met by dietary carbohydrates or via gluconeogenesis, dietary carbohydrate is considered a dispensable, or nonessential, nutrient for adults. An analogy to this would be the nonessential amino acids. These amino acids are just as important to the body for normal endogenous protein synthesis as the 10 essential amino acids but, unlike those, the body is able to make the nonessential amino acids via transamination providing that sufficient substrates are included in the diet.

Cats are carnivores and evolved consuming low carbohydrate diets, so some question if they are able to digest or metabolize dietary carbohydrates. Cats and dogs both lack salivary amylase, the enzyme that can begin the process of digesting carbohydrates. However, both species have sufficient pancreatic amylase as well as intestinal disaccharidases, which allow them to efficiently digest properly processed carbohydrates.[3,5,6,12,13]

There are different forms of dietary carbohydrates, including simple sugars, rapidly digested and slowly digested starches (complex carbohydrates), dietary fibers, and others. Proper processing or cooking is necessary to make starches digestible to mammals, including cats and dogs. In many species, poorly digestible carbohydrates or an overload of simple sugars may induce adverse changes in intestinal metabolism.[14] This also is true for cats given high quantities (25%–40% of the diet) of sugars or raw (indigestible) starch.[15] However, when properly processed complex carbohydrates are provided as a major component of balanced diets (eg, 25%–50% of the diet being dry matter), cats are easily able to digest and use the carbohydrates. In fact, both cats and dogs can digest properly cooked carbohydrates, such as those from grains, with greater than 90% efficiency.[5,6,13]

Post-absorption, both cats and dogs will use the glucose from dietary carbohydrates to help meet their physiologic demand. Studies have shown that cats will increase carbohydrate metabolism, or oxidation, when carbohydrate intake increases and will likewise increase or decrease protein oxidation when intake of that nutrient changes.[16–18] However, having more or less carbohydrate in the diet does not significantly affect gluconeogenesis or blood glucose concentrations in normally fed cats.[19,20]

Grain-free diets are not necessarily low in dietary carbohydrates. Although grains are a common source of dietary carbohydrates, other sources of carbohydrates can include potatoes, beans, tapioca, peas, and other vegetables and fruits. Many grain-free pet foods contain these alternate sources of dietary carbohydrates and may contain at least as much carbohydrate as traditional grain-containing diets. For pet foods that truly are low in carbohydrate, that component of the diet is often replaced with increased dietary fat, which can increase the risk for undesirable weight gain.[21,22]

MEAT OR POULTRY BY-PRODUCTS AND MEALS

Some clients are concerned about the meaning, content, and source of "by-products" from meats or poultry. The lack of understanding may confuse pet owners and lead them to perceive these as poor-quality ingredients.

Meat by-products consist of edible parts and organs such as heart, lungs, stomach, or liver; meat trimmings; bone; and other tissues from mammals, such as cattle or hogs.[23] As defined by AAFCO, by-products do not include hair or hide, horns or hooves, intestinal contents, or feathers from poultry.[23] Compared with skeletal meat alone, by-products actually provide more essential nutrients. For example, meat is lacking in calcium and vitamin A, which are provided in by-products from the bones and liver. Although the components of by-products are not widely consumed by people in the United States, many are considered delicacies for human consumption in other cultures. These also are the same tissues consumed first by animals in the wild.

The "meals" of meat or poultry by-products are created by rendering. Rendering is a cooking process similar to what happens when you boil chicken to separate the broth, fat, and meat for chicken soup. In commercial rendering, fat is separated (and becomes animal fat), and the "soup" is dried to remove the water. The dried product is then ground into a protein-rich powder or meal.[24] Meat meals and poultry meals can provide excellent sources of protein and essential amino acids and can be highly digestible.[25–28] Rendering conditions, as well as the source and handling of raw materials used, can greatly influence the quality of the protein meals produced.[26–28] These variables can affect the protein digestibility of the finished pet food, so pet food companies may contract with specific suppliers to assure the consistent quality of their ingredients. Although detailed information about ingredients may be proprietary, veterinarians can contact the manufacturer to ask about the digestibility of protein in specific pet foods.

Renderers affiliated with USDA-inspected meat or poultry plants will receive animal products only from those facilities, so pet food manufacturers that work exclusively with these renderers will have greater control about the specific content and quality of the by-products that they use. One of the prevailing Internet myths about commercial pet foods states that they may contain rendered remains of pets. It is because of the ability to work with USDA-affiliated renderers that pet food companies can have confidence that their products do not contain dog or cat remains, as has been attested to by members of the Pet Food Institute and confirmed by testing conducted by the USDA's Center for Veterinary Medicine.[29]

Animal Versus Vegetable Source Proteins: Determinants of Protein Quality

The quality of dietary protein is determined by the amino acid composition of the protein, its digestibility, and its ability to meet an animal's amino acid requirements, rather than whether it comes from animal or vegetable sources. Common measures of protein quality are typically conducted on individual sources of protein (ingredients), and use laboratory assays, rodent feeding trials, or both. The associated score generally reflects the amino acid most deficient in that protein, called the "limiting amino acid". For example, soy protein provides at least 100% of most essential amino acids, but it is deficient in methionine and thus receives a lower score based on its methionine content. Used alone, proteins with low scores would provide lower-quality nutrition. Fortunately, the limiting amino acids of different proteins often differ. Complementary proteins are those that provide excess of each other's limiting amino acids so that the combination of ingredients provides all of the necessary amino acids.

By mixing complementary proteins in a diet, the finished product can provide excellent protein quality even though the individual components each have limitations. So although most vegetable source proteins, for example, soy protein, corn gluten meal, or wheat gluten, are incomplete proteins if used alone due to their limiting amino acids, they are highly digestible. When incorporated into a properly cooked diet with complementary proteins, they can contribute to a diet that provides complete, high-quality protein, easily digested by both dogs and cats.

EFFECT OF COOKING ON QUALITY AND DIGESTIBILITY OF NUTRIENTS

Proponents of feeding raw food diets suggest that cooking decreases the nutritional value of meats by decreasing protein digestibility and by destroying enzymes naturally present in foods.

Natural enzymes present in ingredients are proteins and thus cooking temperatures will indeed change their physical properties and deactivate them. However, enzymes in food add very little, if any, value to the digestion processes of dogs and cats. Enzymes in meat and other food ingredients are not specialized digestive enzymes and will not participate in the digestion or assimilation of proteins. Some raw foods contain enzymes that actually serve to inhibit digestion or destroy essential nutrients, such as avidin in raw eggs, thiaminase in fish, and trypsin inhibitory factors in various raw foods. In this case, cooking greatly enhances the nutritional value of the ingredients.[30,31]

Grains and other plant-based ingredients benefit significantly from cooking. Cooking increased the digestibility of the starch from grains between 14% and 208% in multiple studies.[32] Although overcooking can decrease protein digestibility, proper cooking can increase the digestibility of protein from both animal and vegetable sources.[30-34] This is thought to occur due to the physical restructuring or unfolding of proteins during the cooking process, providing more binding sites and making them more susceptible to digestive enzymes and reducing the energy required for digestion.[32,34] Gentle cooking in a microwave did not compromise the digestibility of a raw feline diet and may provide a way to sterilize raw food diets for pets.[35]

About Extrusion Cooking

The effects of cooking on nutrient quality and digestibility can vary with type of cooking method, temperature, time, and amount of moisture.[30,34,36,37] The vast majority of dry foods are cooked using an extrusion process. Extrusion uses a combination of moisture (25%-35%), temperature (100°-150°C), pressure (20-30 bars), and mechanical shear (0.5-5 minutes) to quickly cook the product.[38] Correct extrusion conditions favor higher retention of amino acids, high protein and starch digestibility, decreased lipid oxidation, and higher retention of vitamins.[36] In addition, the extrusion process denatures undesirable enzymes such as antinutritional factors (trypsin inhibitors, haemagglutinins, tannins, and phytates) and sterilizes the finished product.[36] Although overcooking using any method, including extrusion, can decrease the nutritional quality of foods, the relatively high moisture content, moderate temperatures, and short cooking duration help to maintain the nutritional quality of extruded foods.[38]

ADDITIVES AND PRESERVATIVES

Pet owners may be concerned about the list of chemical-sounding names in the ingredient list of pet foods or may have read about "unnecessary additives or preservatives". For these clients, it will be important to help them understand the meaning and use of the "chemicals". It may help to observe a quote from Dr Nathan Myhrvold, shared during televised interview on PBS: "Lots of folks think of this as, 'Oh, my god, there's chemicals in my food!' Well, I'm here to tell you that food is made of chemicals; those chemicals are made of elements; and that's the way it is here on planet Earth. Everything actually is a chemical."[39]

Many of the ingredients listed on pet food labels are vitamins and minerals. Pet owners may not recognize "pyridoxine hydrochloride" as Vitamin B6, "menadione sodium bisulfite complex" as Vitamin K, or "copper proteinate" as a source of essential dietary copper, for example. These are among the 40+ essential nutrients that dogs and cats require and are critical to assure a nutritionally complete and balanced diet.

Other additives may include natural (eg, mixed tocopherols or vitamin E) or synthetic (eg, BHA, TBHQ, ethoxyquin) antioxidant preservatives that function to keep dietary fats and other nutrients stable during storage. Without these antioxidants, the essential fatty acids could become oxidized or rancid and their nutritional value destroyed. Concerns have been raised about the use of chemical or synthetic antioxidants, suggesting that they can be toxic or carcinogenic. Toxicity, for all compounds, is related to dose as well as to route in exposure. For BHA and butylated hydroxytoluene, for example, an extremely high dose can induce adverse effects but the data show they are safe and even suggest they may be anticarcinogenic at lower levels of use.[40–42] As used in pet foods, these antioxidants are safe and are critical to maintain the nutritional value of foods.

SUMMARY

Ingredients are included in diets primarily as a source of nutrients. Animals require specific nutrients, not specific ingredients. Nutritionists and pet food manufacturers formulate diets to provide complete and balanced diets for cats and dogs in various life stages or with different life styles. Ingredients are selected for their nutrient content, as well as their impact on palatability, digestibility, and consumer preferences. The quality of ingredients used is dictated by individual companies working with their suppliers. Unfortunately, indicators of ingredient quality cannot be included on labels, according to regulatory guidelines. The finished product quality depends on selection of ingredients that provide the desired features, as well as the appropriateness of the processing and cooking processes. If veterinarians have questions about the quality of a food, they should contact the manufacturer and inquire about the nutrient profile and the digestibility of the product, which are good markers of the quality of the food. Veterinarians also should consider the history of the company, their pattern of investment into research, and their safety record when considering whether or not to recommend a product.

REFERENCES

1. White PJ, Johnson LA. Corn: chemistry and technology. 2nd edition. St Paul (MN): Am Assoc Cereal Chemists; 2003.
2. Kuhlman G, Laflamme DP, Ballam JM. A simple method for estimating the metabolizable energy content of dry cat foods. Fel Pract 1993;21:16–20.
3. Murray SM, Fahey GC, Merchen NR, et al. Evaluation of selected high-starch flours as ingredients in canine diets. J Anim Sci 1999;77:2180–6.
4. Gajda M, Flickinger EA, Grieshop CM, et al. Corn hybrid affects in vitro and in vivo measures of nutrient digestibility in dogs. J Anim Sci 2005;83:160–71.
5. Carciofi AC, Takakura FS, de-Oliveira LD, et al. Effects of six carbohydrate sources on dog diet digestibility and post-prandial glucose and insulin response. J Anim Physiol Anim Nutr 2008;92:326–36.
6. de-Oliveira LD, Carciofi AC, Oliveira MC, et al. Effects of six carbohydrate sources on diet digestibility and postprandial glucose and insulin responses in cats. J Anim Sci 2008;86:2237–46.

7. Verlinden A, Hesta M, Millet S, et al. Food allergy in dogs and cats: a review. Crit Rev Food Sci Nutr 2006;46:259–73.
8. Garden OA, Pidduck H, Lakhani KH, et al. Inheritance of gluten-sensitivity enteropathy in Irish Setters. Am J Vet Res 2000;61:462–8.
9. Blaza SE, Booles D, Burger IH. Is carbohydrate essential for pregnancy and lactation in dogs?. In: Burger IH, Rivers JP, editors. Nutrition of the dog and cat: Waltham symposium No. 7. Cambridge (United Kingdom): Cambridge University Press; 1989. p. 229–42.
10. Westman E. Is dietary carbohydrate essential for human nutrition? [letter to the editor]. Am J Clin Nutr 2002;75:951–3.
11. Eisert R. Hypercarnivory and the brain: protein requirements of cats reconsidered. J Comp Physiol B 2011;18:1–17.
12. Hore P, Messer M. Studies on disaccharidase activities of the small intestine of the domestic cat and other mammals. Comp Biochem Physiol 1968;24:717–25.
13. Morris JG, Rogers QR. Do cats really need more protein? J Small Anim Pract 1982;23:521–32.
14. Meyer H, Kienzle E. Dietary protein and carbohydrates: relationship to clinical disease. Proceedings of the Purina International Nutrition Symposium. Orlando (FL): Ralston Purina Co; 1991. p. 13–26.
15. Kienzle E. Blood sugar levels and renal sugar excretion after the intake of high carbohydrate diets in cats. J Nutr 1994;124:2563S–7S.
16. Russell K, Murgatroyd PR, Batt RM. Net protein oxidation is adapted to dietary protein intake in domestic cats (Felis silvestris catus). J Nutr 2002;132:456–60.
17. Russell K, Lobley GE, Millward DJ. Whole-body protein turnover of a carnivore, Felis silvestris catus. Br J Nutr 2003;89:29–37.
18. Green AS, Ramsey JJ, Villaverde C, et al. Cats are able to adapt protein oxidation to protein intake provided their requirement for dietary protein is met. J Nutr 2008;138:1053–60.
19. Hoenig M, Jordan ET, Glushka J, et al. Effects of macronutrients, age, and obesity on 6- and 24-h postprandial glucose metabolism in cats. Am J Physiol Regul Integr Comp Physiol 2011;301:R1798–807.
20. Thiess S, Becskei C, Tomsa K, et al. Effects of high carbohydrate and high fat diet on plasma metabolite levels and on IV glucose tolerance test in intact and neutered male cats. J Feline Med Surg 2004;6:207–18.
21. Nguyen PG, Dumon HJ, Siliart BS, et al. Effects of dietary fat and energy on body weight and composition after gonadectomy in cats. Am J Vet Res 2004;65:1708–13.
22. Backus RC, Cave NJ, Keisler DH. Gonadectomy and high dietary fat but not high dietary carbohydrate induce gains in body weight and fat of domestic cats. Br J Nutr 2007;98:641–50.
23. Association of American Feed Control Officials. Official publication 2013. Champaign, IL: Association of American Feed Control Officials, Inc; 2013.
24. Thompson A. Ingredients: where pet food starts. Top Companion Anim Med 2008;23:127–32.
25. Murray SM, Patil AR, Fahey GC, et al. Raw and rendered animal by-products as ingredients in dog diets. J Anim Sci 1997;75:2497–505.
26. Johnson ML, Parsons CM, Fahey GC, et al. Effects of species raw material source, ash content, and processing temperature on amino acid digestibility of animal by-product meals by cecectomized roosters and ileally cannulated dogs. J Anim Sci 1998;76:1112–22.
27. Shirley RB, Parsons CM. Effect of ash content on protein quality of meat and bone meal. Poultry Sci 2001;80:626–32.

28. Wang X, Parsons CM. Effect of raw material source, processing systems, and processing temperatures on amino acid digestibility of meat and bone meals. Poultry Sci 1998;77:834–41.

29. Myers MJ, Farrell DE, Heller DN, et al. Development of a polymerase chain reaction-based method to identify species-specific components in dog food. Am J Vet Res 2004;65:99–103.

30. Zhang Y, Parsons CM, Weingartner KE, et al. Effects of extrusion and expelling on the nutritional quality of conventional and Kunitz trypsin inhibitor-free soybeans. Poult Sci 1993;72:2299–308.

31. Evenepoel P, Geypens B, Luypaerts A, et al. Digestibility of cooked and raw egg protein in humans as assessed by stable isotope techniques. J Nutr 1998;128: 1716–22.

32. Carmody RN, Wrangham RW. The energetic significance of cooking. J Hum Evol 2009;57:379–91.

33. Boback SM, Cox CL, Ott BD, et al. Cooking and grinding reduces the cost of meat digestion. Comp Biochem Physiol A Mol Integr Physiol 2007;148:651–6.

34. Bax ML, Aubry L, Ferreira C, et al. Cooking temperature is a key determinant of in vitro meat protein digestion rate: investigation of underlying mechanisms. J Agric Food Chem 2012;60:2569–76.

35. Kerr KR, Vester Voler BM, Morris CL, et al. Apparent total tract energy and macro-nutrient digestibility and fecal fermentative end-product concentrations of do-mestic cats fed extruded, raw beef-based, and cooked beef-based diets. J Anim Sci 2012;90:515–22.

36. Singh S, Gamlath S, Wakeling L. Nutritional aspects of food extrusion: a review. Int J Food Sci Tech 2007;42:916–29.

37. Santé-Lhoutellier V, Astruc T, Marinova P, et al. Effect of meat cooking on physi-ochemical state and in vitro digestibility of myofibrillar proteins. J Agric Food Chem 2008;56:1488–94.

38. Sorensen M. A review of the effects of ingredient composition and processing conditions on the physical qualities of extruded high-energy fish feed as measured by prevailing methods. Aquaculture Nutr 2012;18:233–48.

39. Hamilton D, Sweet J. "NOVA: Can I eat that?" aired on NOVA on PBS channels. Transcript. WGBH Educational Foundation. 2012. Available at: http://www.pbs.org/wgbh/nova/body/can-i-eat-that.html. PBS airdate October 31, 2012.

40. Moch RW. Pathology of BHA- and BHT-induced lesions. Food Chem Toxicol 1986; 24:1167–9.

41. Tobe M, Furuya T, Kawasaki Y, et al. Six-month toxicity study of butylated hydrox-yanisole in beagle dogs. Food Chem Toxicol 1986;24:1223–8.

42. Williams GM, Iatropoulos MJ, Whysner J. Safety assessment of butylated hydrox-yanisole and butylated hydroxytoluene as antioxidant food additives. Food Chem Toxicol 1999;37:1027–38.

Macronutrients in Feline Health

Cecilia Villaverde, BVSc, PhD[a],*, Andrea J. Fascetti, VMD, PhD[b]

KEYWORDS

- Feline • Protein • Fat • Carbohydrates • Nutrition

KEY POINTS

- The ideal dietary macronutrient composition to optimize health in cats is still undetermined.
- Studies on feral cat prey and colony cats' preferences suggest that high-protein, high-fat, and very-low-carbohydrate diets are preferentially selected.
- High-protein diets (>40% protein calories) are beneficial for the management of weight loss in cats, and high-protein diets may also help geriatric cats maintain muscle mass.
- Ad libitum consumption of high-fat, and not high-carbohydrate diets, is associated with weight gain.
- Macronutrient modification in feline diets is helpful to manage a variety of diseases, such as obesity, diabetes mellitus (DM), liver disease, lower urinary tract disease, and renal disease, among others; however, the evidence for a particular macronutrient distribution beyond providing minimal requirements for the prevention of most of these diseases is lacking.

INTRODUCTION

Currently there is tremendous interest in identifying the ideal macronutrient profile to maximize health and longevity in cats. Current nutritional recommendations[1,2] are based on minimal intake data rather than optimal intake. Minimal requirements are established with easily measured outcomes, such as growth or adequate reproductive performance. Optimal intake is harder to measure, because defining and measuring health and longevity outcomes is not an easy task.

Some investigators have suggested that the carbohydrate content of commercial, dry cat foods is too high and, simultaneously, the protein content too low for a strict carnivore, such as cats, and they have hypothesized that several chronic diseases in this species, in particular obesity and DM,[3,4] could be related to feeding dry foods. There is no clear evidence, however, supporting this statement.

Disclosures: C. Villaverde and A.J. Fascetti consult for various pet food companies.
[a] Departament de Ciència Animal i dels Aliments (Animal and Food Science Department), Universitat Autònoma de Barcelona, Edifici V, Campus UAB, Bellaterra 08193, Spain; [b] Department of Molecular Biosciences, University of California Davis, One Shields Avenue, Davis, CA 95616-8741, USA
* Corresponding author.
E-mail address: cecilia.villaverde@uab.cat

Vet Clin Small Anim 44 (2014) 699–717
http://dx.doi.org/10.1016/j.cvsm.2014.03.007
0195-5616/14/$ – see front matter © 2014 Elsevier Inc. All rights reserved.

MACRONUTRIENT REQUIREMENTS FOR CATS: MINIMUMS AND MAXIMUMS

The 3 macronutrients in foods are protein, fat, and carbohydrates. These are called macronutrients because they are present in high amounts in the diet (compared with vitamins and minerals, the micronutrients) and provide energy.[1] Fat provides more than twice the metabolizable energy (ME) of protein and carbohydrates (**Table 1**). In the United States, the guaranteed analysis on cat food labels provides the minimum value on an as-fed basis for crude protein and crude fat, but carbohydrates are not required to be reported. The carbohydrate content of a diet can be estimated by a calculated difference (100 − [crude protein + crude fat + moisture + ash + crude fiber]), but this value is an estimate at best.

Protein Requirements

Protein, in addition to providing energy, is a source of nitrogen and essential amino acids. The current minimal protein requirement for adult cat foods is reported to be 50 to 65 g/1000 kcal ME (**Table 2**).[1,2] This is assumed to provide 2.3 to 5.2 g protein/kg body weight. The Association of American Feed Control Officials' (AAFCO) recommendations are higher than the National Research Council's (NRC) to account for individual variation and assumed differences in bioavailability and digestibility between commercial and experimental diets. Dry commercial feline diets generally have a crude protein content of 30% to 40% on an ME basis, whereas canned and raw foods are generally higher in protein.

In addition to meeting nitrogen requirements, feline diets also have to provide essential amino acids above their respective minimal requirements. Cats require 11 essential amino acids: methionine, lysine, threonine, tryptophan, histidine, leucine, isoleucine, valine, arginine, phenylalanine, and taurine.[1] Taurine is a β-sulfonic amino acid that is not incorporated into proteins.[5] If essential amino acid requirements are not met, the diet is inadequate, irrespective of the total amount of protein.

Protein requirements in cats are considerably higher than in dogs. This has been attributed to the fact that protein catabolic enzymes are not down-regulated in this carnivorous species.[6,7] Recent research has shown that cats can adapt protein oxidation to their protein intake[8,9] but only if this intake is above their minimal requirement.[9] Cats' inability to down-regulate their hepatic catabolic capacity at low protein intakes may only partially explain this carnivore's high nitrogen requirement. A second, emerging argument suggests that cats have evolved a high capacity for gluconeogenesis from amino acids to solve the dilemma of how to survive on a high-protein, prey-based diet as a small mammal with a large brain,[10] given the reliance of brain tissue on glucose for energy. Although arguably this overarching model[10] requires more direct

Table 1
Estimated crude and metabolizable energy content (based on modified Atwater factors) of protein, fat, and carbohydrates in commercial cat food

Macronutrient	Crude Energy (kcal/g)	Metabolizable Energy (kcal/g)[a]
Protein	5.7	3.5
Fat	9.4	8.5
Carbohydrates (nitrogen-free extract)	4.1	3.5

[a] Modified Atwater factors assume fixed macronutrient digestibilities and thus are useful only to provide a ballpark approximation to the energy density of a diet.
Data from National Research Council. Nutrient requirements of dogs and cats. Washington, DC: The National Academies Press; 2006.

Table 2
Protein and fat requirements for adult cats at maintenance

		Diet (Dry Matter), g/kg	Metabolizable Energy, g/1000 kcal	Metabolic Body Weight, g/kg$^{0.67}$
Protein	NRC	200	50	4.96
	AAFCO	260	65	Not available
Fat	NRC	90	22.5	2.2
	AAFCO	90	22.5	Not available

Data from National Research Council. Nutrient Requirements of Dogs and Cats. Washington, DC: The National Academies Press; 2006; and AAFCO. Official Publication. Oxford (IN): Association of American Feed Control Officials; 2008.

scientific support, the hypotheses and ideas are intriguing and provide a platform for future studies.

Classical research regarding minimum protein and amino acid requirements in cats has been done using growth studies and, in adults, nitrogen balance studies,[11] and these have been the basis for the NRC[1] and AAFCO[2] to establish their minimum protein requirements. Nitrogen balance studies are based on feeding diets with differing protein levels and measuring nitrogen intake and excretion. When the nitrogen balance is negative, protein intake is considered inadequate or losses excessive. This method is time consuming and can be inexact for several reasons, such as underestimating nitrogen excretion.[12] More recently, it has been suggested that nitrogen balance may not be the best method to assess protein requirements, because cats can maintain a zero nitrogen balance in the face of inadequate protein intake.[13] A recent study fed adult cats 3 different dietary protein concentrations for 2 months. The minimum protein intake to maintain a zero nitrogen balance was determined to be 2.1 g/kg$^{0.75}$, whereas the amount of protein to maintain lean body mass (LBM) was estimated to be higher, at 7.8 g/kg$^{0.75}$. The investigators concluded that using other outcomes, such as the maintenance of adequate muscle mass, might be a more appropriate determinant of protein requirements.[13]

The clinical signs of overt protein and amino acid deficiencies include lack of growth, decrease in food intake, muscle wasting, hypoalbuminemia, skin alterations, a decrease in essential plasma amino acid concentrations, and other signs.[1,14–16] Protein calorie malnutrition in humans is associated with increased morbidity and mortality.[17–19] The effect on health and longevity of marginal protein intakes over long periods of time is unknown in cats.[3]

Regarding maximal allowances, neither the NRC[1] or the AAFCO[2] established a maximum level for protein or amino acids in the diet of adult cats, although safe upper limits exist for required amino acids for growth. A safe upper limit is the highest level of a daily nutrient intake that has been proved safe, and it has not been set for protein because there are no data reported on adverse effects associated with high-protein intakes. As discussed previously, cats are metabolically prepared to eat and metabolize high- and very-high-protein meals, yet there are some diseases where high-protein diets are contraindicated, such as renal disease[20] and urate urolithiasis.[21]

Fat Requirements

The need for dietary fat comes from the requirement for essential fatty acids, although dietary fat is important by itself as a concentrated energy source and contributes to palatability. Commercial feline diets often have a crude fat content of 30% to 40% on an ME basis, but it can be higher, especially in canned or raw foods. The minimum fat requirements reported by NRC and AAFCO are 22.5 g/1000 kcal ME (see **Table 2**).[1,2] Mammals can synthesize saturated and monounsaturated fatty acids de novo from glucose.[1] Polyunsaturated fatty acids (PUFAs) from the omega-3 and -6 families, however, cannot be synthesized by mammals and need to be provided by the diet.[22]

The 18 carbon precursors of the omega-3 and -6 families are α-linolenic acid (C18:3ω3) and linoleic acid (C18:2ω6). Most mammals can elongate and further desaturate these fatty acids to obtain longer-chain omega-3 and -6 PUFAs (**Fig. 1**).[23,24] In cats, however, the activity of the enzyme Δ6 desaturase, although present,[25] is low; thus, longer-chain PUFAs, such as arachidonic acid (C20:4ω6), could be considered essential in cats, especially during reproduction and growth.[1,26] There is no clear evidence at this time that longer-chain omega-3 PUFAs (eicosapentaenoic acid [C20:5ω3] and docosahexaenoic acid [C22:6ω3]) are required by cats.

The major signs of essential fatty acid deficiency are dermatologic due to the role of linoleic acid in maintaining skin barrier function.[27] Typical signs are dry coat and dandruff.[1] Other signs include fatty liver and infertility in female cats.[28,29] In puppies, it has been shown that omega-3 PUFAs are important for brain and retinal development[30] but there are no data to support that this applies to kittens at this time.

The NRC[1] has defined a safe upper limit for total fat (82.5 g/1000 kcal, 330 g/kg of dry matter), linoleic acid (13.8 g/1000 kcal, 55 g/kg of dry matter), and arachidonic acid (0.5 g/1000 kcal, 2 g/kg of dry matter). The total dietary fat maximum value (equivalent to approximately 70% fat ME) is considerably higher than what is present in the average feline maintenance diet. The fat content in the latter ranges between 30% and 40% ME but can be higher (up to 60% ME) in some canned and raw diets. This safe upper limit has been established as a precaution rather than due to specific reported adverse effects; such high-fat diets would make it impossible to provide other essential nutrients (such as protein) in sufficient amounts Similarly, the safe upper limit for both linoleic and arachidonic acids are for precaution and no adverse effects of their excess have been described in cats.

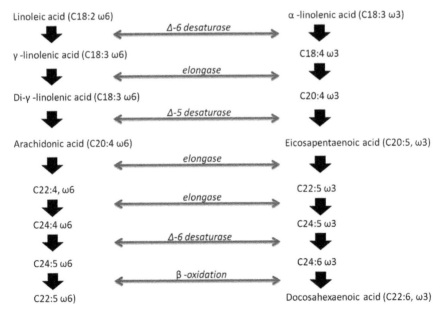

Fig. 1. Metabolism of essential fatty acids from the omega-6 and omega-3 families.

Carbohydrate Requirements

Carbohydrate is not an essential dietary nutrient for cats. It provides energy and glucose, which is metabolically essential, and can be either obtained by dietary carbohydrate or synthesized in the body from amino acids or glycerol (via gluconeogenesis).[31] Glucose has several functions in the body, such as being a critical energy source for cells and a precursor for many important substances, such as vitamin C and fatty acids. There are no minimal requirements established for this macronutrient. Carbohydrate in commercial diets is provided between 0% (some canned and raw diets) and 50% ME.

Carbohydrate metabolism in cats is different from that of omnivores, such as dogs. Although cats lack salivary amylase[32] and they have lower amounts of pancreatic amylase compared with dogs,[33] they can digest starch well, in particular when processed and cooked.[34] It has been suggested that the intestinal transport of sugar to the enterocyte does not adapt to varying concentrations of dietary carbohydrate intake.[35] Vomiting and diarrhea have been described in cats fed high amounts of sugar[36] and starch,[36,37] but not all studies feeding high carbohydrate diets have seen this.[9] Cats have low glucokinase activity in their liver.[38,39] Glucokinase has a low binding affinity for glucose and phosphorylates it when concentrations are elevated. They instead have hexokinase, an enzyme that has a high binding affinity for glucose, and phosphorylates it when present in low concentrations. This can result in a slower rate of clearance of glucose in the face of a high-carbohydrate meal.

These specific metabolic differences of the carbohydrate metabolism of cats could be the result from evolutionary adaptation to eating low-carbohydrate diets as prey.[7] Despite these adaptations, cats can digest, absorb, and use carbohydrates obtained from the diet, in the amounts commonly used in commercial feline foods (20%–40% ME). The eating behavior of cats, which favors small frequent feedings[40] over 1 or 2 large meals, results in a lower intake of carbohydrates per meal and seems well handled by its enzymatic systems.

MACRONUTRIENT PREFERENCES OF CATS

One recent study evaluated the preferences of cats for combinations of different foods (using the same ingredients and texture) varying in their macronutrient content.[41] The findings suggested that depending on the choices provided, cats may select a diet with a low-carbohydrate content and thus high in protein and high in fat. In this study, the cats tended to choose a diet with a caloric distribution of 52% protein, 36% fat, and 12% carbohydrates on an ME basis (**Fig. 2**), independent of the physical form of the diet. The investigators hypothesized that there is actually a carbohydrate ceiling of 70 kcal per day that the cats do not willingly exceed. This represents 20% to 30% of ME for 3- to 5-kg cats. If true, this ceiling might result in marginal intakes of energy and protein when cats are offered very-high-carbohydrate diets.

The investigators justify this ceiling due to suggested metabolic limitations of cats. The limitations alluded to, however, such as limited ability to digest and metabolize carbohydrate, have not been supported by evidence. Preference studies are complex and aspects besides macronutrient composition (such as ingredients used, processing, and texture) may play an important role as well. One retrospective study[42] summarized the findings of 27 studies that reported body composition of typical prey for cats (small mammals and birds). Such studies should be interpreted with caution, because purpose-bred animals are frequently used to estimate the nutrient content of prey, and their actual body composition can be different. There was tremendous variation on how the data were reported and the methods used to determine body

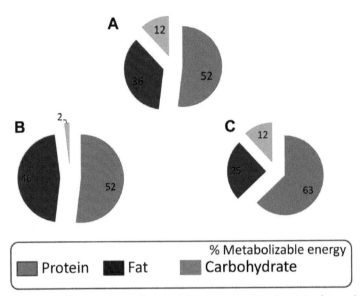

Fig. 2. Caloric distribution (on an ME basis) of the macronutrient (protein, fat, and carbohydrate) content of preferred diet composition in a study evaluating preferences of colony cats (*A*) and average of prey species from a review study (*B*) and from wild caught prey in Northern California (*C*). (*Data from* Refs.[41–43])

composition of the prey species. The average caloric distribution of the prey reported in this study (52%, 46%, and 2% ME of protein, fat, and carbohydrates, respectively) (see **Fig. 2**), was similar to the macronutrient profile preferred by colony cats in the study from Hewson-Hughes colleagues,[41] particularly with regard to protein content. One study analyzing wild prey of cats in Northern California[43] noted that wild animals are usually leaner and have more mineral content than their purpose-bred counterparts, especially rats. This study found an estimated average composition of typical feline prey to be 63% protein, 25% fat, and 12% carbohydrate on an ME basis (see **Fig. 2**). Although higher in protein than the 2 previously cited studies, there seems to be a general agreement among the articles that the natural diet of cats is low in carbohydrates, is high in protein, and has a variable content of fat.

Prey studies give insight into the diet feral cats have available and have evolved eating; however, there is no evidence to suggest feral cats eating prey have a longer life span or live healthier lives in association with this type of diet. Thus, these studies cannot be a basis to establish optimal macronutrient intakes to maximize health and longevity.

MACRONUTRIENTS AND AGE

The digestion and absorption of macronutrients, specifically protein and fat, decline as cats age, particularly in those over 12 years.[44–48] Several studies have demonstrated no significant difference in orocecal transit times in young compared with older cats.[49,50] One study reported a positive correlation between fat digestibility and serum vitamin E concentrations.[44] This same study also reported a positive correlation between fat and protein digestibility and plasma vitamin B_{12} concentrations.[44]

In humans, sarcopenia (muscle mass loss associated with aging[51]) is common and has been associated with increased morbidity and mortality.[52] This syndrome is multifactorial and has not been studied extensively in veterinary medicine[53] but it is receiving increasing attention. One small pilot study[54] evaluated muscle mass using ultrasound and CT imaging in aged (greater than 8 years old) and adult (less than 5 years old) Labrador retrievers and reported that the older dogs had a lower mean epaxial muscle area. More recently researchers have evaluated body composition of geriatric cats compared with adults. Using dual energy x-ray absorptiometry (DEXA), the investigators reported that there was a decrease in LBM over time.[55] This could be due, in part, to the reported decrease in the digestibility of dietary protein. These findings imply that geriatric cats may have a higher protein requirement than adults. Laflamme and Hannah[13] estimated the theoretic daily protein requirement of cats at different ages to maintain LBM using DEXA and reported that it increased markedly with age, from 4.17 g protein/kg body weight at 8 years of age to 11.12 g protein/kg body weight at 16 years. The investigators suggest that maintaining LBM in aged cats at the same level as adults may not be a realistic goal, even when cats are consuming a high-protein diet. This is because LBM loss associated with aging likely depends on other factors in addition to protein intake and digestibility. Taken together, these results suggest that protein in feline geriatric diets should not be decreased compared with adult maintenance diets, and there may be a benefit in feeding a diet with higher protein content.

Weight loss is also common in geriatric cats (as opposed to adult and mature cats, where obesity is more of a problem).[46,56] As a consequence of the lower fat digestibility, these animals also have a lower energy digestibility, resulting in an increase in their apparent ME needs.[56] The ME of a diet is closely related to its fat content, due to fat's high energy density. High amounts of highly digestible and palatable fat may be indicated in the diets for geriatric cats, to compensate for its lower digestibility. The high prevalence of low digestibility of fat might indicate, however, that the other macronutrients (protein and carbohydrate), although less energy dense, could be better energy sources. Additional studies are warranted.

MACRONUTRIENTS AND MAINTAINING A HEALTHY BODY WEIGHT

Obesity and overweightedness are common problems in cats, with an estimated prevalence in the United States ranging between 29[57] and 35%,[58] although many experts suspect it may be higher. Reported risk factors[57-61] include age, gender, underestimation of body condition score by owners, and sterilization status. Thus, middle-aged castrated male cats with owners not aware of the problem are at high risk. Other suggested risk factors, but not identified in all studies, are indoor living,[57] ad libitum feeding,[61] and the use of dry premium high-fat foods.[57,58] Obesity is a concern due to its association with several health problems, such as skin disease, DM, and hepatic lipidosis.[57,58]

The traditional approach to maintaining a lean body weight in most species has been to use diets with a low energy density to facilitate energy restriction.[62] The macronutrient composition can be altered to achieve this low energy density and the historical recommendation has been to use low-fat, high-fiber diets. Fiber is very low in energy density (nutritionists assume that it provides few to no calories) and provides bulk and volume to the diet. Fiber can potentially improve satiety, as has been reported in dogs,[63] but research in cats is lacking.

The Role of Protein

In recent years, there has been increasing interest and research regarding the role of protein in weight loss in humans. It is believed that high-protein diets in humans can have positive effects by promoting satiety, increasing thermogenesis, sparing LBM during weight loss, and perhaps even helping to prevent weight regain.[64–67] Most of the studies are short term (months); thus, the long-term effects of such diets are still unknown. It is hard to identify what is more important: an increase in protein intake or a concurrent decrease in carbohydrate intake. Because calories can only come from the 3 macronutrients, studies that assess different protein intakes usually substitute protein for carbohydrate, making separating the effects of each macronutrient difficult. One study[68] compared 4 diets in overweight people: high protein–low carbohydrate (20% and 25% ME, respectively), high protein–normal carbohydrate (20% and 50% ME), normal protein–low carbohydrate (10% and 25% ME), and normal protein–normal carbohydrate (10% and 50% ME). All patients lost weight successfully, eating restricted amounts of the 4 diets, but the 2 groups consuming the high-protein diets had a greater degree of weight loss. This result suggests that, at least in humans, the beneficial effect of these diets on weight loss is attributable to the high protein content rather than the low carbohydrate intake. As for prevention of weight gain, research is scarce and very short term, although some studies suggest these diets can potentially be helpful in humans.[69,70] In cats, high-protein diets have shown benefits during weight loss, but as described later, the data do not fully support a weight prevention role for this macronutrient when high-protein diets are fed at will.

Satiety

Overall, the research regarding high-protein diets and weight loss in humans has reported that there are no marked differences compared with the traditional approach of calorie restriction when the tested diets are fed in restricted amounts. Alternatively, the consumption of a high-protein (25%–30% ME) diet results in loss of weight and fat mass when consumed ad libitum compared with a higher-carbohydrate, lower-protein diet (15% ME).[64,65] These findings spurred the hypothesis that the consumption of high-protein diets in humans promotes a reduction in voluntary food intake compared with lower-protein diets.

One recent study[69] offered normal weight or slightly overweight individuals a moderate-protein, high-fat diet (15% protein and 35% fat ME) for 2 weeks and then an isocaloric, high-protein, and lower-fat diet (30% and 20% ME, respectively) for 2 more weeks, and individuals reported a decrease in hunger. Afterward participants were offered the high-protein diet ad libitum and the individuals lost weight, voluntarily eating less, without any changes in energy expenditure. In another study,[70] lean and overweight patients were fed ad libitum for 12 weeks with 3 different isocaloric diets containing 5%, 15%, and 30% protein (ME) in substitution for carbohydrates. Although all subjects lost weight, they did not report any differences in hunger or fullness. The energy deficit (intake minus expenditure), however, was higher in the high-protein treatment group, a finding that prompted the investigators to suggest that protein content of a diet might be more important than energy in driving food intake.

It has also been suggested that amino acids can affect appetite-regulating hormones or that the increase in oxygen consumption and body temperature associated with protein metabolism might contribute to a satiety effect.[65] These studies have several limitations, such as their short-term duration and variations in the overall nutrient content of the test diets.

Comparatively, there is a paucity of research in cats. One recent study[71] compared the effect of the 3 macronutrients fed as a bolus (maltodextrin, lard, and canned chicken) or combined into 3 dry extruded diets (high fat, 53% ME fat; high protein, 50% ME protein; and high carbohydrate, 47% ME carbohydrate) on the appetite regulatory hormones (insulin, ghrelin, and leptin). Ghrelin is a fast-acting orexigenic hormone[72] that increases in periods of hunger, whereas leptin is anorexigenic and long acting, increasing in association with a decrease in energy intake.[73] The concentration of leptin is proportional to body fat mass in several species, including cats.[74,75] The maltodextrin bolus increased blood glucose and insulin concentrations, but there was no effect on ghrelin and leptin concentrations measured up to 6 hours after a meal. The protein load suppressed ghrelin to a lesser extent than the other nutrients. When the dry, extruded diets were meal-fed twice daily for 2 weeks, there were no differences in insulin, ghrelin, or leptin concentrations. This report suggests that protein does not promote satiety more than the other macronutrients, a finding contrary to what has been suggested in humans,[76] although reported results are conflicting.[77,78]

Several studies comparing high- and low-protein diets in cats fed ad libitum have not shown a decrease in voluntary food and energy intake in cats, rather the contrary. One short-term study[79] fed lean cats 2 diets differing in protein content (51.9% vs 35.3% ME) ad libitum and found a trend toward a higher energy intake in the high-protein diet treatment group (despite this diet being less calorically dense). A medium-term study,[80] following lean female cats 6 months postovariohysterectomy, reported a trend toward higher food and energy intake in cats eating a high-protein diet (45.7% ME) compared with a moderate-protein diet (32.4% ME). In this study, the high-protein diet had a higher energy density. Coradini and colleagues[37] fed lean cats 2 isocaloric diets, one high in protein (47% ME) and the second low in protein (21% ME). Cats were energy restricted the first 4 weeks and then fed ad libitum for 8 weeks. When fed ad libitum, cats eating the high-protein diet ate more and subsequently gained more weight. A study in obese cats fed isocaloric diets containing protein at either 27.1% or 47.3% of the calories for 4 months found that the obese cats ate more when offered the high-protein diet.[81] These investigators hypothesized that protein palatability could promote food intake and might be an evolutionary advantage for cats.

The intrinsic limitation of these studies is that the specific influence of each macronutrient on the observed response cannot be separated. Also, the diets among the different studies differ in energy density, processing, ingredients, texture, feeding method, and so forth. In any case, with the current information available, there does not seem to be a clear strong effect of high-protein diets on satiety in cats.

Thermogenesis

The energy content of food is reported as ME, which is the energy available for metabolic reactions and is calculated as the gross energy of food minus the energy lost in the feces and urine.[1] The difference between ME and net energy (energy that is deposited in the body) is heat production, also called thermogenesis. It has been shown that protein consumption might result in higher food-induced thermogenesis (the heat loss associated with digestion and metabolism of food) compared with fat and carbohydrates.[82] This means that protein provides less net energy than carbohydrate, despite providing the same ME.

It has been suggested that the relative inefficiency of protein might be due to the cost of protein turnover, gluconeogenesis, and urea synthesis[64]; however, the overall effect on daily energy expenditure is considered small. Researchers have estimated that increasing protein consumption from 15% to 30% ME in humans increases energy expenditure by only 23 kcal.[64] The significance of such slight increases over time is unknown. One study[83] found that postprandial heat production in lean cats was higher when fed a high-protein diet (41.7% ME) compared with cats fed a lower-protein diet (26.5%). Some indirect data may provide further insight.

In obese cats undergoing weight loss, 2 studies have investigated energy expenditure in diets with varying protein concentrations. Nguyen and colleagues[84] fed 2 diets providing protein at 40.4% and 50.5% of the calories and found no effect of diet on resting energy expenditure during weight loss. Laflamme and Hannah[85] evaluated different protein concentrations (36.5% vs 46.4% ME) in cats during weight loss. They did not find any difference in the energy intake needed to achieve a desirable rate of weight loss, but they did not measure energy expenditure, so it can be concluded that, if there was any effect on thermogenesis, it was small. Alternatively, a study[86] conducted in obese cats during weight loss reported a positive effect of consuming a high-protein diet (41.5% ME) compared with a moderate-protein diet (31.1% ME) regarding the energy needed to achieve weight loss. Cats fed the high-protein diet required less calorie restriction during weight loss. After weight loss, both groups were placed on the high-protein diet for the weight maintenance phase. The cats that lost weight with the high-protein diet also maintained their body weight with more calories compared with the moderate-protein group.

Short-term studies[9,79] in lean cats fed varying concentrations of dietary protein did not report any difference in energy expenditure measured by calorimetry. Longer-term studies report either no effect or a mild effect of protein on energy expenditure.[83,87] Contrary to the previous studies, Wei and colleagues[81] demonstrated that obese cats fed a 47.3% protein (ME) diet had a higher energy expenditure than cats fed the lower-protein diet (27.1% ME). Taken together, consumption of high-protein diets potentially results in diet-induced thermogenesis, but it is likely that the effect is so small that the current measuring techniques (indirect calorimetry) fail to detect it.

Lean body mass preservation
There is general agreement that high-protein diets during weight loss result in more fat mass and less LBM loss.[85,86] This is considered a healthy way to lose weight. A high loss of LBM during weight reduction may result in an overall lower energy expenditure (fat is less metabolically active than muscle) and may predispose individuals to weight regain and the yo-yo dieting phenomena.

As with any effect of protein intake in lean individuals, the results are conflicting. Short-term studies[9,79] have not found any effect of varying protein concentrations on body composition. In a 6-month study from Nguyen and colleagues,[87] lean neutered cats were fed 1 of 2 isocaloric diets, containing a different amount of protein calories (27% or 46.5% ME) to maintain body weight. Cats fed the lower-protein diet not only lost weight during the study but also lost LBM. Cats consuming the 46.5% protein diet maintained body weight and gained LBM. Alternatively, in a second study where sterilized female cats were fed ad libitum moderate- or high-proteins diets (32.4% or 45.7% protein ME, respectively), no differences in body composition were reported between the groups.[80] Similar outcomes were reported when the same diets used in the aforementioned study were fed to growing kittens.[88] Thus, at this time, it does not seem that a high-protein diet (greater than 40% ME) has any beneficial effects on body composition in lean adult cats compared with diets providing at least 32% protein calories.

Weight Gain: Fat or Carbohydrates?

In recent years, some investigators have proposed that the high carbohydrate content of dry cat foods has caused an increase in feline obesity,[3,4] yet data to support this hypothesis are lacking. On the contrary, retrospective and prospective studies have emerged to challenge this hypothesis. In 1 study, colony cats[89] were fed semipurified diets ad libitum for 13 weeks before and 17 weeks after gonadectomy. The cats were fed 1 of 4 semipurified diets, substituting fat for carbohydrate to provide 9%, 25%, 44%, and 64% of the ME in a diet with a constant protein:ME ratio. Only cats consuming the highest-fat dietary treatment gained weight prior to gonadectomy. Postgonadectomy, all cats gained weight, but weight gain was positively correlated to fat inclusion and negatively correlated with carbohydrate inclusion in the diet. One study of feeding-restricted amounts of a moderate-protein, high-carbohydrate diet (47.8% ME) compared with a higher-protein, lower-carbohydrate diet (23.1% ME) resulted in weight loss.[87] Another study[37] reported that feeding a higher-protein, moderate-carbohydrate diet (23% ME) compared with a lower-protein, higher-carbohydrate diet (51% ME), both with equal concentrations of dietary fat, resulted in weight gain when fed ad libitum for 8 weeks. Finally, a recently published prospective survey study specifically tested the hypothesis that an increase in feeding energy-dense, premium diets to cats was associated with a change in the prevalence of obesity in that population since it was last surveyed 15 years before.[59] Despite an increased proportion of owners feeding dry food daily since the last survey, the lack of association with dry food feeding and the absence of an increase in obesity over the study period did not support the hypothesis that energy-dense dry food feeding increases the risk of feline obesity. In the model used by the investigators, only 3 variables were significant: owner underestimation of the cat's body condition, the leg length of the cat, and the cat's age. The investigators concluded that more effort should be placed in educating owners to what a normal body type is for a cat rather than changing feeding patterns or food type.

Together these results suggest that high-carbohydrate diets are not associated with weight gain and obesity in cats, but that other factors (such as dietary fat, energy density, and feeding method) may play a more important role.

MACRONUTRIENTS AND PREVENTION OF DISEASES: WHAT IS THE EVIDENCE?
Diabetes Mellitus

In cats, DM is frequently associated with insulin resistance rather than with a lack of insulin production. Historically, nutritional management in cats with DM was extrapolated from human medicine and consisted of feeding diets with a high-fiber content and the inclusion of complex carbohydrates.[90] Fiber, due to its effects on overall diet digestibility, can result in a lower blood glucose postprandial peak and slower and more constant glucose absorption. There is currently only 1 study evaluating the effects of dietary fiber on naturally occurring diabetes in cats.[91] Cats in this randomized crossover study were fed either a diet containing 12% cellulose (insoluble fiber, DM; 19% of total dietary fiber) or low insoluble fiber (4.1% total dietary fiber) for 24 weeks. Mean preprandial glucose concentrations, most postprandial glucose concentrations, and 12-hour mean glucose concentrations were significantly lower in the cats eating the high-insoluble-fiber diet. The carbohydrate content was higher in the low-fiber diet. The investigators could not rule out the possibility that the higher cornstarch content in the low-fiber diet may have had an impact on glycemic control in this study.

Over the past decade, research has emerged evaluating the use of low-carbohydrate diets (high-fat, moderate to high in protein, approximately 40% protein calories) in the management of this disease.[92] There have been 4 clinical trials in diabetic cats investigating the potential benefits of feeding low-carbohydrate, high-protein diets. The first clinical trial[93] examined the use of a high-protein canned diet (Purina Veterinary Diets DM Dietetic Management Feline Formula) in 9 cats for 3 months. All of the cats were initially adapted to a high-fiber, moderate-fat canned diet (Hill's Prescription Diet w/d Feline) for a standardization period of 1 month prior to the study. The cats remained stable on the high-protein canned diet and most owners thought their cats were more active. In 3 cats, insulin was discontinued all together, although serum fructosamine concentrations increased in these cats. There was no diet effect on serum glucose concentrations. The study was conducted for only 3 months, with no long-term follow-up on the cats.

A second study evaluated 18 cats fed a high-protein diet (Hill's Science Diet Feline Growth, canned) and a hypoglycemic agent, acarbose.[94] Cats were classified as responders (insulin discontinued) and nonresponders (continued to require insulin or glipizide). Eleven of 18 cats were discontinued from insulin by the end of the 4-month study. Overall, responders lost weight during the study and nonresponders had significantly less body fat than cats that did respond. Both responders and nonresponders had similar decreases in serum glucose and fructosamine concentrations.

A third study[95] compared cats fed either a high-fiber diet (Hill's Prescription Diet w/d Feline, canned) or a high-protein, low-carbohydrate diet (Hill's Science Diet Feline Growth, canned) for 4 months. More cats fed the low-carbohydrate diet (12/13) had reduced fructosamine and glucose concentrations compared with the cats (3/9) eating the high-fiber diet. The cats consuming the high-protein, low-carbohydrate diet also, however, lost weight during the study. Food intake data were not collected, so it is difficult to determine if weight loss was the result of a reduction in calories, an effect of diet, or a reduction or discontinuation in the insulin dose.

A fourth study found no difference in improvement rates between the groups of cats fed therapeutic lower-carbohydrate diets (Purina Veterinary Diets DM Dietetic Management Feline Formula, canned) and those fed dry and canned maintenance diets (Pro Plan Adult Cat Total Care Chicken & Rice Formula, Nestlé Purina PetCare, and Friskies Special Diet Turkey & Giblets Dinner for Adult Cats, Nestlé Purina PetCare),[96] although the experimental diet group showed lower fructosamine levels. This study also reported a gain in body weight in cats in both dietary groups.

It is difficult to discern from this research which nutrient modifications are having a positive impact. Most published studies tested commercially available products rather than evaluating particular nutrients. Such an approach precludes conclusions about the impact of a particular nutrient. There seems to be some clear evidence that supplementation with insoluble fiber helps reduce the glycemic response and assists in managing diabetic patients. The results of carbohydrate restriction or protein augmentation are less clear. With respect to the research in cats, the amount of protein fed in some of the studies is no higher than many other diets on the market. Another challenge with interpreting the literature is that the carbohydrate concentrations of the test diets in these studies ranged between 5% and 12% ME, but there are no dose-response studies on increasing levels of carbohydrates in cats with DM. One finding that does recur throughout the studies is that overweight or obese diabetic patients that lose weight develop better control or in some cases revert to a nondiabetic state. This finding suggests that in obese or overweight cats, weight loss to achieve an ideal body condition may be the most effective modification toward achieving better glycemic control or in cats reverting to a nondiabetic state.

The positive response in a subset of feline patients with DM to low-carbohydrate (below 15% ME)/high-fat (above 40% ME)/moderate–high protein (approximately 40% ME) diets has triggered interest in determining if feeding this type of diet can prevent this disease from appearing in the first place. Is feeding a high-carbohydrate diet a risk factor for DM in cats? Some investigators have suggested that consumption of high-carbohydrate diets can result in pancreatic β-cell exhaustion, secondary to higher blood glucose peak concentrations, leading to insulin resistance and DM.[4] A recent review by Verbrugghe and colleagues[31] concludes that the evidence again is weak and conflicting.

Some studies have documented that high-carbohydrate diets (ranging from 32% to 51% ME) can result in higher glucose and insulin concentrations in healthy cats.[37,97,98] One recent study[71] found, however, that a high-carbohydrate dry diet (compared with high-protein and high-fat diets) increased the glucose response but not the insulin response. A second study reported that a high-fat diet (compared with a high-carbohydrate diet) resulted in a reduction in glucose clearance.[98] Epidemiologic analysis has found no association between the feeding of dry foods and the development of DM in cats. Two recent population studies further refute the hypothesis that feeding dry-type extruded diets long-term are the cause of diabetes in cats.[99,100] In studies comparing different diets in lean and obese cats, it can be seen that the effect of being obese is much more marked than the effect of the dietary macronutrient composition.[83,101,102] And, as discussed previously, low-carbohydrate diets are more likely to result in obesity when free-fed than typical dry food.

Chronic Kidney Disease

Diet therapy is the cornerstone of medical management of cats with chronic kidney disease (CKD). Dietary modifications typically recommended for cats with this condition include a reduction in protein (between 22% and 28% ME) and sodium, alkalinization, phosphorus restriction, and supplementation with potassium, B vitamins, and omega-3 fatty acids.[20]

In laboratory animals, it has been described that dietary protein restriction can slow down progression of CKD by reducing renal blood flow, glomerular filtration rate, and proteinuria.[103] In cats, there is general agreement that the use of protein and phosphorus-restricted diets in these patients can improve quality of life by reducing clinical signs[104] but there is not clear evidence that protein affects progression.[105,106] Research in cats with spontaneous CKD, however, is scarce and there is still some controversy surrounding this issue.

Despite the positive effect of renal diets in the treatment of CKD, there is no evidence at this time that it has any effect in the prevention of CKD or even that high-protein diets are deleterious to feline kidneys. Some diets for senior cats are formulated to provide protein close to the minimal recommendation established by AAFCO[2] (at or below 30% ME), and one of the stated reasons by the product manufacturers is to avoid overtaxing the kidneys. Although it is true that CKD is the most common disease in geriatric cats[107] and that it is usually diagnosed when there is advanced kidney damage, feeding apparently healthy older cats as if they have some degree of renal dysfunction is not justified by existing scientific evidence. Alternatively, it may even be contraindicated, given the risk of muscle wasting and loss of LBM in older cats. Thus, at this time, there is no reason to recommend reducing protein intake in cats that have not been diagnosed with CKD.

SUMMARY

The ideal dietary macronutrient profile for cats is currently unknown. The natural diet of feral cats is low in carbohydrates, high in protein, and with a variable content of fat. At this time, however, there is not enough evidence to support that feeding such a diet or any diet with a specific macronutrient profile results in longer, healthier lives for all cats. Moreover, there are no scientific data to support that typical commercial dry maintenance diets are the cause of chronic disease in this species. Taken together, the data support the idea that there is not one ideal diet for all cats, and different strategies might be better suited to individual animals. Nutritional recommendations should be tailored to each cat based on age, body condition, and the presence of disease.

REFERENCES

1. National Research Council. Nutrient requirements of dogs and cats. Washington, DC: The National Academies Press; 2006.
2. AAFCO. Official publication. Oxford (IN): Association of American Feed Control Officials; 2008.
3. Zoran DL, Buffington CA. Effects of nutrition choices and lifestyle changes on the well-being of cats, a carnivore that has moved indoors. J Am Vet Med Assoc 2011;239:596–606.
4. Rand JS, Fleeman LM, Farrow HA, et al. Canine and feline diabetes mellitus: nature or nurture? J Nutr 2004;134:S2072–80.
5. Earle KE, Markwell PJ. Taurine: an essential nutrient for the cat. A brief review of the biochemistry of its requirement and the clinical consequences of deficiency. Nutr Res 1995;15:53–8.
6. Rogers QR, Morris JG, Freedland RA. Lack of hepatic enzymatic adaptation to low and high levels of dietary protein in the adult cat. Enzyme 1977;22:348–56.
7. Morris JG. Idiosyncratic nutrient requirements of cats appear to be diet induced evolutionary adaptations. Nutr Res Rev 2002;15:153–68.
8. Russell K, Lobley GE, Millward DJ. Whole-body protein turnover of a carnivore, Felis silvestris catus. Br J Nutr 2003;89:29–37.
9. Green AS, Ramsey JJ, Villaverde C, et al. Cats are able to adapt protein oxidation to protein intake provided their requirement for dietary protein Is met. J Nutr 2008;138:1053–60.
10. Eisert R. Hypercarnivory and the brain: protein requirements of cats reconsidered. J Comp Physiol B 2011;181:1–17.
11. Tome D. Criteria and markers for protein quality assessment - a review. Br J Nutr 2012;108:S222–9.
12. Hegsted DM. Balance studies. J Nutr 1976;106:307–11.
13. Laflamme DP, Hannah SS. Discrepancy between use of lean body mass or nitrogen balance to determine protein requirements for adult cats. J Feline Med Surg 2013;15:691–7.
14. Morris JG, Rogers QR. Ammonia intoxication in the near-adult cat as a result of a dietary deficiency of arginine. Science 1978;199:431–2.
15. Pion PD, Kittleson MD, Rogers QR, et al. Myocardial failure in cats associated with low plasma taurine: a reversible cardiomyopathy. Science 1987;237:764–8.
16. Yu S, Rogers QR, Morris JG. Effect of low levels of dietary tyrosine on the hair colour of cats. J Small Anim Pract 2001;42:176–80.
17. Sam J, Nguyen GC. Protein-calorie malnutrition as a prognostic indicator of mortality among patients hospitalized with cirrhosis and portal hypertension. Liver Int 2009;29:1396–402.
18. Collins N. Nutrition and wound healing: strategies to improve patient outcomes. Wounds 2004;16:S12–8.
19. Crogan NL, Pasvogel A. The influence of protein-calorie malnutrition on quality of life in nursing homes. J Gerontol A Biol Sci Med Sci 2003;58:159–64.
20. Elliott DA. Nutritional management of chronic renal disease in dogs and cats. Vet Clin North Am Small Anim Pract 2006;36:1377–84.
21. Bartges JW, Kirk CA. Nutrition and lower urinary tract disease in cats. Vet Clin North Am Small Anim Pract 2006;36:1361–76.
22. Bézard J, Blond JP, Bernard A, et al. The metabolism and availability of essential fatty acids in animal and human tissues. Reprod Nutr Dev 1994;34:539–68.

23. Dunbar BL, Bigley KE, Bauer JE. Early and sustained enrichment of serum n-3 long chain polyunsaturated fatty acids in dogs fed a flaxseed supplemented diet. Lipids 2010;45:1–10.
24. Nakamura MT, Nara TY. Essential fatty acid synthesis and its regulation in mammals. Prostaglandins Leukot Essent Fatty Acids 2003;68:145–50.
25. Pawlosky R, Barnes A, Salem N. Essential fatty acid metabolism in the feline: relationship between liver and brain production of long-chain polyunsaturated fatty acids. J Lipid Res 1994;35:2032–40.
26. Bauer JE. Metabolic basis for the essential nature of fatty acids and the unique dietary fatty acid requirements of cats. J Am Vet Med Assoc 2006;229:1729–32.
27. Elias PM, Brown BE, Ziboh VA. The permeability barrier in essential fatty acid deficiency: evidence for a direct role for linoleic acid in barrier function. J Invest Dermatol 1980;74:230–3.
28. MacDonald ML, Rogers QR, Morris JG, et al. Effects of linoleate and arachidonate deficiencies on reproduction and spermatogenesis in the cat. J Nutr 1984; 114:719–26.
29. MacDonald ML, Rogers QR, Morris JG. Effects of dietary arachidonate deficiency on the aggregation of cat platelets. Comp Biochem Physiol C 1984;78:123–6.
30. Bauer JE. Responses of dogs to dietary omega-3 fatty acids. J Am Vet Med Assoc 2007;231:1657–61.
31. Verbrugghe A, Hesta M, Daminet S, et al. Nutritional modulation of insulin resistance in the true carnivorous cat: a review. Crit Rev Food Sci Nutr 2012;52: 172–82.
32. Morris JG, Trudell J, Pencovic T. Carbohydrate digestion by domestic cat (Felis Catus). Br J Nutr 1977;37:365–73.
33. McGeachin RL, Akin JR. Amylase levels in the tissues and body fluids of the domestic cat (Felis catus). Comp Biochem Physiol B 1979;63:437–9.
34. Kienzle E. Carbohydrate metabolism of the cat 1. Activity af amylase in the gastrointestinal tract of the cat. J Anim Physiol Anim Nutr 1993;69:92–101.
35. Buddington RK, Chen JW, Diamond JM. Dietary regulation of intestinal brush-border sugar and amino acid transport in carnivores. Am J Physiol 1991;261: R793–801.
36. Kienzle E. Carbohydrate metabolism of the cat 2. Digestion of the starch. J Anim Physiol Anim Nutr 1993;69:102–14.
37. Coradini M, Rand JS, Morton JM, et al. Effects of two commercially available feline diets on glucose and insulin concentrations, insulin sensitivity and energetic efficiency of weight gain. Br J Nutr 2011;106:S64–77.
38. Hiskett EK, Suwitheechon OU, Lindbloom-Hawley S, et al. Lack of glucokinase regulatory protein expression may contribute to low glucokinase activity in feline liver. Vet Res Commun 2009;33:227–40.
39. Tanaka A, Inoue A, Takeguchi A, et al. Comparison of expression of glucokinase gene and activities of enzymes related to glucose metabolism in livers between dog and cat. Vet Res Commun 2005;29:477–85.
40. Kane E, Rogers Q, Morris J. Feeding behavior of the cat fed laboratory and commercial diets. Nutr Res 1981;1:499–507.
41. Hewson-Hughes AK, Hewson-Hughes VL, Miller AT, et al. Geometric analysis of macronutrient selection in the adult domestic cat, Felis catus. J Exp Biol 2011; 214:1039–51.
42. Plantinga EA, Bosch G, Hendriks WH. Estimation of the dietary nutrient profile of free-roaming feral cats: possible implications for nutrition of domestic cats. Br J Nutr 2011;106:S35–48.

43. Kremen NA, Calvert CC, Larsen JA, et al. Body composition and amino acid concentrations of select birds and mammals consumed by cats in northern and central California. J Anim Sci 2013;91:1270–6.

44. Patil AR, Cupp CJ. Addressing age-related changes in feline digestion. In: Nestlé Purina Companion Animal Nutrition Summit, Focus on Gerontology. Clearwater Beach (FL): 2010. p. 55–61.

45. Taylor EJ, Adams C, Neville R. Some nutritional aspects of ageing in dogs and cats. Proc Nutr Soc 1995;54:645–56.

46. Perez-Camargo G. Cat nutrition: what's new in the old? Compend Contin Educ Pract Vet 2004;26:5–10.

47. Teshima E, Brunetto MA, Vasconcellos RS, et al. Nutrient digestibility, but not mineral absorption, is age-dependent in cats. J Anim Physiol Anim Nutr 2010; 94:251–8.

48. Peachey SE, Dawson JM, Harper EJ. The effect of ageing on nutrient digestibility by cats fed beef tallow-, sunflower oil- or olive oil-enriched diets. Growth Dev Aging 1999;63:61–70.

49. Papasouliotis K, Sparkes AH, Gruffydd-Jones TJ, et al. Use of the breath hydrogen test to assess the effect of age on orocecal transit time and carbohydrate assimilation in cats. Am J Vet Res 1998;59:1299–302.

50. Peachey SE, Dawson JM, Harper EJ. Gastrointestinal transit times in young and old cats. Comp Biochem Physiol A Mol Integr Physiol 2000;126:85–90.

51. Doherty TJ. Invited review: aging and sarcopenia. J Appl Physiol (1985) 2003; 95:1717–27.

52. Baumgartner RN, Koehler KM, Gallagher D, et al. Epidemiology of sarcopenia among the elderly in New Mexico. Am J Epidemiol 1998;147:755–63.

53. Freeman LM. Cachexia and sarcopenia: emerging syndromes of importance in dogs and cats. J Vet Intern Med 2012;26:3–17.

54. Hutchinson D, Sutherland-Smith J, Watson AL, et al. Assessment of methods of evaluating sarcopenia in old dogs. Am J Vet Res 2012;73:1794–800.

55. Cupp CJ, Jean-Philippe C, Kerr WW, et al. Effect of nutritional interventions on longevity of senior cats. Int J Appl Res Vet Med 2007;5:133–49.

56. Laflamme DP. Nutrition for aging cats and dogs and the importance of body condition. Vet Clin North Am Small Anim Pract 2005;35:713–42.

57. Scarlett JM, Donoghue S, Saidla J, et al. Overweight cats: prevalence and risk factors. Int J Obes Relat Metab Disord 1994;18:S22–8.

58. Lund EM, Armstrong PJ, Kirk CA, et al. Prevalence and risk factors for obesity in adult cats from private US Veterinary Practices. Int J Appl Res Vet Med 2005;3: 88–96.

59. Cave NJ, Allan FJ, Schokkenbroek SL, et al. A cross-sectional study to compare changes in the prevalence and risk factors for feline obesity between 1993 and 2007 in New Zealand. Prev Vet Med 2012;107:121–33.

60. Colliard L, Paragon BM, Lemuet B, et al. Prevalence and risk factors of obesity in an urban population of healthy cats. J Feline Med Surg 2009;11:135–40.

61. Russell K, Sabin R, Holt S, et al. Influence of feeding regimen on body condition in the cat. J Small Anim Pract 2000;41:12–7.

62. Michel KE. Nutritional management of body weight. In: Fascetti AJ, Delaney SJ, editors. Applied veterinary clinical nutrition. Chichester (United Kingdom): Wiley-Blackwell; 2012. p. 109–24.

63. Bosch G, Verbrugghe A, Hesta M, et al. The effects of dietary fibre type on satiety-related hormones and voluntary food intake in dogs. Br J Nutr 2009; 102:318–25.

64. Halton TL, Hu FB. The effects of high protein diets on thermogenesis, satiety and weight loss: a critical review. J Am Coll Nutr 2004;23:373–85.

65. Te Morenga L, Mann J. The role of high-protein diets in body weight management and health. Br J Nutr 2012;108:S130–8.

66. Westerterp-Plantenga MS, Lejeune MP, Nijs I, et al. High protein intake sustains weight maintenance after body weight loss in humans. Int J Obes Relat Metab Disord 2004;28:57–64.

67. Paddon-Jones D, Westman E, Mattes RD, et al. Protein, weight management, and satiety. Am J Clin Nutr 2008;87:S1558–61.

68. Soenen S, Bonomi AG, Lemmens SG, et al. Relatively high-protein or "low-carb" energy-restricted diets for body weight loss and body weight maintenance? Physiol Behav 2012;107:374–80.

69. Weigle DS, Breen PA, Matthys CC, et al. A high-protein diet induces sustained reductions in appetite, ad libitum caloric intake, and body weight despite compensatory changes in diurnal plasma leptin and ghrelin concentrations. Am J Clin Nutr 2005;82:41–8.

70. Martens EA, Lemmens SG, Westerterp-Plantenga MS. Protein leverage affects energy intake of high protein diets in humans. Am J Clin Nutr 2013;97:86–93.

71. Deng P, Ridge TK, Graves TK, et al. Effects of dietary macronutrient composition and feeding frequency on fasting and postprandial hormone response in domestic cats. J Nutr Sci 2013;2:e36.

72. Meier U, Gressner AM. Endocrine regulation of energy metabolism: review of pathobiochemical and clinical chemical aspects of leptin, ghrelin, adiponectin, and resistin. Clin Chem 2004;50:1511–25.

73. Klok MD, Jakobsdottir S, Drent ML. The role of leptin and ghrelin in the regulation of food intake and body weight in humans: a review. Obes Rev 2007;8: 21–34.

74. Appleton DJ, Rand JS, Sunvold GD. Plasma leptin concentrations in cats: reference range, effect of weight gain and relationship with adiposity as measured by dual energy X-ray absorptiometry. J Feline Med Surg 2000;2:191–9.

75. Martin L, Siliart B, Dumon H, et al. Leptin, body fat content and energy expenditure in intact and gonadectomized adult cats: a preliminary study. J Anim Physiol Anim Nutr 2001;85:195–9.

76. Lejeune MP, Westerterp KR, Adam TC, et al. Ghrelin and glucagon-like peptide 1 concentrations, 24-h satiety, and energy and substrate metabolism during a high-protein diet and measured in a respiration chamber. Am J Clin Nutr 2006;83:89–94.

77. Smeets AJ, Soenen S, Luscombe-Marsh ND, et al. Energy expenditure, satiety, and plasma ghrelin, glucagon-like peptide 1, and peptide tyrosine-tyrosine concentrations following a single high-protein lunch. J Nutr 2008;138:698–702.

78. Erdmann J, Lippl F, Schusdziarra V. Differential effect of protein and fat on plasma ghrelin levels in man. Regul Pept 2003;116:101–7.

79. Russell K, Murgatroyd PR, Batt RM. Net protein oxidation is adapted to dietary protein intake in domestic cats (Felis silvestris catus). J Nutr 2002;132:456–60.

80. Vester BM, Sutter SM, Keel TL, et al. Ovariohysterectomy alters body composition and adipose and skeletal muscle gene expression in cats fed a high-protein or moderate-protein diet. Animal 2009;3:1287–98.

81. Wei A, Fascetti AJ, Liu KJ, et al. Influence of a high-protein diet on energy balance in obese cats allowed ad libitum access to food. J Anim Physiol Anim Nutr 2011;95:359–67.

82. Westerterp KR. Diet induced thermogenesis. Nutr Metab (Lond) 2004;1:5.

83. Hoenig M, Thomaseth K, Waldron M, et al. Insulin sensitivity, fat distribution, and adipocytokine response to different diets in lean and obese cats before and after weight loss. Am J Physiol Regul Integr Comp Physiol 2007;292: R227–34.
84. Nguyen P, Dumon H, Martin L, et al. Weight loss does not influence energy expenditure or leucine metabolism in obese cats. J Nutr 2002;132:S1649–51.
85. Laflamme DP, Hannah SS. Increased dietary protein promotes fat loss and reduces loss of lean body mass during weight loss in cats. Int J Appl Res Vet Med 2005;3:62–8.
86. Vasconcellos RS, Borges NC, Gonc KN, et al. Protein intake during weight loss influences the energy required for weight loss and maintenance in cats. J Nutr 2009;139:855–60.
87. Nguyen P, Leray V, Dumon H, et al. High protein intake affects lean body mass but not energy expenditure in nonobese neutered cats. J Nutr 2004;134: S2084–6.
88. Vester BM, Belsito KR, Swanson KS. Serum metabolites, ghrelin and leptin are modified by age and/or diet in weanling kittens fed either a high- or moderate-protein diet. Anim Sci J 2012;83:426–33.
89. Backus RC, Cave NJ, Keisler DH. Gonadectomy and high dietary fat but not high dietary carbohydrate induce gains in body weight and fat of domestic cats. Br J Nutr 2007;98:641–50.
90. Nelson RW. Dietary management of diabetes mellitus. J Small Anim Pract 1992; 33:213–7.
91. Nelson RW, Scott-Moncrieff JC, Feldman EC, et al. Effect of dietary insoluble fiber on control of glycemia in cats with naturally acquired diabetes mellitus. J Am Vet Med Assoc 2000;216:1082–8.
92. Kirk CA. Feline diabetes mellitus: low carbohydrates versus high fiber? Vet Clin North Am Small Anim Pract 2006;36:1297–306.
93. Frank G, Anderson W, Pazak H. Use of a high-protein diet in the management of feline diabetes mellitus. Vet Ther 2001;2:238–46.
94. Mazzaferro EM, Greco DS, Turner AS, et al. Treatment of feline diabetes mellitus using an alpha-glucosidase inhibitor and a low-carbohydrate diet. J Feline Med Surg 2003;5:183–9.
95. Bennett N, Greco DS, Peterson ME, et al. Comparison of a low carbohydrate-low fiber diet and a moderate carbohydrate-high fiber diet in the management of feline diabetes mellitus. J Feline Med Surg 2006;8:73–84.
96. Hall TD, Mahony O, Rozanski EA, et al. Effects of diet on glucose control in cats with diabetes mellitus treated with twice daily insulin glargine. J Feline Med Surg 2009;11:125–30.
97. Farrow HA, Rand JS, Morton JM, et al. Effect of dietary carbohydrate, fat, and protein on postprandial glycemia and energy intake in cats. J Vet Intern Med 2013;27:1121–35.
98. Thiess S, Becskei C, Tomsa K, et al. Effects of high carbohydrate and high fat diet on plasma metabolite levels and on i.v. glucose tolerance test in intact and neutered male cats. J Feline Med Surg 2004;6:207–18.
99. McCann TM, Simpson KE, Shaw DJ, et al. Feline diabetes mellitus in the UK: the prevalence within an insured cat population and a questionnaire-based putative risk factor analysis. J Feline Med Surg 2007;9:289–99.
100. Slingerland LI, Fazilova VV, Plantinga EA, et al. Indoor confinement and physical inactivity rather than the proportion of dry food are risk factors in the development of feline type 2 diabetes mellitus. Vet J 2009;179:247–53.

101. Hoenig M, Jordan ET, Glushka J, et al. Effect of macronutrients, age, and obesity on 6- and 24-h postprandial glucose metabolism in cats. Am J Physiol Regul Integr Comp Physiol 2011;301:R1798–807.
102. Kley S, Hoenig M, Glushka J, et al. The impact of obesity, sex, and diet on hepatic glucose production in cats. Am J Physiol Regul Integr Comp Physiol 2009; 296:R936–43.
103. Lentine K, Wrone EM. New insights into protein intake and progression of renal disease. Curr Opin Nephrol Hypertens 2004;13:333–6.
104. Elliott J, Rawlings JM, Markwell PJ, et al. Survival of cats with naturally occurring chronic renal failure: effect of dietary management. J Small Anim Pract 2000;41: 235–42.
105. Adams LG, Polzin DJ, Osborne CA, et al. Influence of dietary protein/calorie intake on renal morphology and function in cats with 5/6 nephrectomy. Lab Invest 1994;70:347–57.
106. Finco DR, Brown SA, Brown CA, et al. Protein and calorie effects on progression of induced chronic renal failure in cats. Am J Vet Res 1998;59:575–82.
107. Bartges JW. Chronic kidney disease in dogs and cats. Vet Clin North Am Small Anim Pract 2012;42:669–92.

Nutrition for Working and Service Dogs

Joseph Wakshlag, DVM, PhD[a],*, Justin Shmalberg, DVM[b]

KEYWORDS

- Nutrition • Glycolysis • Fat • Protein • Glycogen repletion • Omega-3 fatty acids

KEY POINTS

- Sprinting dogs require a balanced moderate protein, fat, and carbohydrate diet for optimal performance.
- Endurance dogs (hunting and patrol dogs working more than 1.5–2 hours a day) require higher-fat diets to fuel mitochondrial biogenesis and to enhance oxidative phosphorylation capacity.
- High-intensity repeated exercise over a moderate duration (ie, agility and field trial/hunt test dogs) benefits from postexercise carbohydrate supplementation.
- The geriatric athlete with degenerative joint disease should receive supplemental dietary long-chain omega-3 fatty acids.

INTRODUCTION

Conformation, genetics, and behavioral drive are the major determinants of success in canine athletes, although controllable variables, such as training and nutrition, play an important role. The scope and breadth of canine athletic events has expanded dramatically in the past 30 years, but with limited research on performance nutrition. However, there are considerable data examining nutritional physiology in endurance dogs (eg, sled dogs) and in sprinting dogs (eg, racing greyhounds). Nutritional studies for more popular canine activities, such as agility, field trial, and detection, are rare. Therefore, application of translational principles from sled dogs and greyhounds to such activities is necessary. This article highlights basic nutritional physiology and interventions for exercise, and reviews newer investigations regarding aging working and service dogs, and canine detection activities.

THE ENERGETIC COST OF ACTIVITY

Exercise principally relies on ATP derived from the use of substrates, such as carbohydrate, protein, or fat. The energetic potential of a diet is commonly reported in

[a] Department of Clinical Sciences, College of Veterinary Medicine, Cornell University, VMC 1-120 Box 34, Ithaca, NY 14853, USA; [b] Department of Clinical Sciences, University of Florida, 2015 SW 15th Street, Gainesville, FL 32610, USA
* Corresponding author.
E-mail address: dr.joesh@gmail.com

Vet Clin Small Anim 44 (2014) 719–740
http://dx.doi.org/10.1016/j.cvsm.2014.03.008
0195-5616/14/$ – see front matter © 2014 Elsevier Inc. All rights reserved.
vetsmall.theclinics.com

kilocalories (kcal) or kilojoules (kJ). Kilocalories, also referred to as calories, are equivalent to 4.16 kJ in the metric system. Metabolizable energy (ME), as reported on pet food labels, refers to the dietary energy remaining after factoring in energy lost in urine, feces, and gases. Current pet food regulations use the modified Atwater factors to estimate food energy, which assigns protein and carbohydrate an ME value of 3.5 kcal/g, and fat a value of 8.5 kcal/g.[1,2] However, the actual ME is principally determined by dietary fat, and by total dietary fiber content of a diet.[2] Because fiber not only dilutes calories in foods but also affects absorption of nutrients, it is not usually a significant concern when feeding athletic dogs, as little is incorporated into performance rations. Feeding trials are used to directly calculate the energetic potential of any given diet and are considered the gold standard.[2]

The National Research Council (NRC) has established energy requirements for dogs based on the available scientific literature.[2] A multiplication factor is applied to the exponential equation for metabolic body weight (MBW = [kg body weight]$^{0.75}$) to determine the energy expenditure of dogs in different conditions. The NRC estimates that active pet dogs require 130 × MBW kcal/d for maintenance energy requirements (MERs).[2] Overall, the active dog will typically require this amount of energy and, depending on the daily activity, these energy requirements will increase. In general, this can be minimally a 5% to 10% increase from the MER, as observed in greyhounds, up to an eightfold increase observed in racing endurance sled dogs. The effects of increasing physical activity and of training during treadmill exercise have been extensively studied in dogs. Such studies use indirect calorimetry, which determines caloric expenditure by measuring the rate of oxygen consumption. The maximum oxygen consumption during exercise (VO$_2$ max) reflects the maximal energy that can be generated via oxygen utilization in the mitochondrial electron transport chain; hence, is a direct correlation to the energy that can be generated for muscle activity. An average 20-kg foxhound or Alaskan sled dog working near VO$_2$ max requires approximately 700 to 900 kcal per hour of work based on the experimental conditions set forth in simulated treadmill exercise.[3–5] This caloric expenditure during exercise is directly related to the distance traveled. Therefore, the expected caloric needs for canine activities should be proportional to the distance of that activity, not the intensity of the exercise (**Table 1**). For example, whippet racing would

Table 1
The integrative energetic cost of selected common canine activities

Low (<25% Increase)[a]	Moderate	High (>100% Increase)[a]
Agility	Bikejoring (2–10 mi)	Sled dog racing (>20 mi)
Obedience or conformation	Carting (2–10 mi)	Bikejoring (>10 mi)
Disc dog	Field trials	Carting (>10 mi)
Dock jumping	Herding	Hunting (>3 h)
Greyhound racing	Hunting (<3 h)	
Earthdog	Search and rescue	
Low-activity service	Weight pulling	
Coursing	Sled dog racing (<20 mi)	
Flyball	High-activity service	

[a] The exercise amounts for many of these activities have not been reported. In general, short periods of activity, even if vigorous, have small effects on caloric requirements. The moderate and high categories depend greatly on the distance traveled and the ambient temperature. This is based on typical active dog lifestyle maintenance energy requirements of 132 (kg)$^{0.75}$.

be expected to require less caloric expenditure as compared with field trials, which cover longer distances.

Both maximal oxygen consumption and endurance are directly related to skeletal muscle mitochondrial density and volume. However, there are many other factors to take into consideration during canine performance, such as ambient temperature, thermal stress (mitigated by panting), and variability in terrain, including slope.[6] Treadmill exercise with an incline decreases the efficiency of energy use and increases caloric expenditure because of the need for vertical rise. It has been hypothesized that larger dogs exert more energy to accommodate for the gravitational fall that occurs on decline.[4,5,7,8] Uneven footing or poor footing (snow and sand), as well as load bearing, also result in increased energy expenditure.[9]

Field studies examining energy expenditure of racing greyhounds have shown that the average 32- to 35-kg greyhound expends approximately 2050 to 2160 kcal (150–160 kcal/kg$^{0.75}$) per day for typical training activities, which is only slightly elevated from active dog maintenance energy values.[10,11] As the distance traveled per day in racing greyhounds is relatively short, this comparatively high MER for the limited activity may be a reflection of the increased muscle-to–fat mass ratio of greyhounds, rather than increased activity. Hill and colleagues[11] also suggest that feed restriction during racing from the normal daily intake of approximately 155 kcal/kg$^{0.75}$ to a restricted intake of only 137 kcal/kg$^{0.75}$ decreased racing times, suggesting that mild caloric restriction may provide performance advantages, at least in sprinters. Of course, this type of feed restriction would occur only for the 1 or 2 days of eventing, with resumption of normal feeding patterns after the event.

Numerous studies have examined the caloric needs of sled dogs during long-distance exercise. Daily caloric requirements have ranged from 228 kcal/kg$^{0.75}$ to 1052 ± 192 kcal/kg$^{0.75}$ body weight per day,[12,13] with the latter study being in extremely cold conditions over mountainous terrain with dogs running more than 12 hours per day.[14] These endurance sled dogs, which weighed on average 24 kg, would need to consume approximately 10,000 kcal per day to maintain their body weight in these conditions. Many dogs in such conditions use body reserves of lipids and amino acids to meet the caloric demands, as practical limits to food intake impair caloric consumption.

Studies of modest endurance activity suggest that an average medium-sized hunting dog with a body weight between 15 and 30 kg working approximately 3 hours in cooler climates would expend approximately 281 kcal/kg$^{0.75}$ per day, which is roughly double the NRC MER, which is consistent with the intermediate distance traveled.[15] The increased MER during such activities may not be recognized by owners, making underfeeding a potential issue during multiple-day events. Reciprocally, some owners may feed excessively, particularly treats, during a competition. Extra feeding and treat consumption should be taken into consideration as part of the daily caloric intake, particularly for agility and other speed-dependent activities where overfeeding can lead to need for defecation and increased fecal mass, which can effect event performance.

ENERGY AND DEMAND: FAT AND CARBOHYDRATE

The respiratory quotient (RQ) is the ratio of CO_2 production divided by oxygen consumption, and is generally measured using indirect calorimetry in laboratory studies. If the RQ is close to 0.7, fat is likely the primary energetic substrate (fat contains more carbon than other metabolic fuels). An RQ closer to 1 suggests glucose metabolism. Amino acid oxidation results in an RQ between that required to burn fat or carbohydrate (approximately 0.8). Early in exercise, generally within the first 20 to 30 minutes, protein oxidation is minimal, and therefore substrate use and changes in oxygen consumption can be examined when feeding diets differing in only carbohydrate and fat.[16]

Multiple studies have investigated energy intensity and duration as related to VO_2 max and RQ values.[17,18] These foundational studies suggest that dogs exercising at 40% of their VO_2 max, or 40% of maximal aerobic exercise, primarily use fat for energy. Exercise at 30% to 70% of VO_2 max relies on a mixture of glucose and fatty acid catabolism. An animal reaching 70% or higher of maximal oxygen consumption, as is common in sprinting athletes, primarily relies on glucose for energy, and therefore displays an RQ closer to 1.[16,19,20]

Animals performing at maximal speed during the first few seconds of exercise quickly deplete small ATP reserves and then use easily accessible energy from the phospho-creatine system that generates ATP through shuttling inorganic phosphate to ADP via creatine-phosphate stored in muscle. Prolonged exercise of high intensity then uses glycogenolysis (generation of glucose from glycogen), which subsequently generates energy through anaerobic glycolysis for a few minutes, generating ATP from pyruvate via the citric acid cycle. However, if the pyruvate cannot be fed into the citric acid cycle, then lactic acid is formed and can lead to pH changes and intracellular dysfunction.

Carbohydrate oxidation becomes a major source of energy for long-term exercise at greater than 50% of maximal oxygen consumption (20 minutes–2 hours) as long as sufficient glycogen is present for glycogenolysis and the rate of conversion of pyruvate to acetyl-CoA is adequate. Some protein oxidation and gluconeogenesis will take place if glycogen is depleted in endurance exercise, and the dog will subsequently be unable to sustain oxygen consumption above 50% to 60% of VO_2 max for extended periods.

Fatty acid oxidation begins within minutes, but does not peak until approximately 30 minutes of exercise and sustains an oxygen consumption rate between 30% and 50% of the maximum. Oxidation of fatty acids provides acetyl-CoA for the citric acid cycle at a constant rate, which allows some dogs to exercise at this low to moderate oxygen consumption for multiple hours with minimal fatigue.[16,21,22] Dogs display higher concentrations of type I (low myosin ATPase) and Type IIa (aerobic) muscle fibers than other species, such as the cat, which permits these higher rates of aerobic metabolism, especially from fatty acids.[23,24]

The time to exhaustion during low-intensity exercise in dogs does not correlate to glycogen depletion,[25] unlike in humans, who use carbohydrate loading to increase stamina.[26] The generation of energy from fat allows consumption of over 70% of the ME intake during long-duration low-intensity to moderate-intensity exercise, suggesting a propensity for fat utilization that may be due to the dog's aforementioned high aerobic activity in skeletal muscle and to an increased mitochondrial density as compared with humans.[27] Kronfeld and colleagues[28] showed that dogs perform equally well on diets containing almost no carbohydrate (1 g/1000 kcal) as compared with 2 diets with increasing carbohydrate content in moderate-intensity working sled dogs.[29] All diets contained elevated amounts of protein for gluconeogenesis as well. Interestingly, endurance huskies racing approximately 160 km per day over 5 days showed immediate glycogen depletion followed by an increase in skeletal muscle glycogen and a gradual depletion of skeletal muscle triglyceride over many days of running. This provides further support for the adaptation of dogs to fat utilization, which spares muscle glycogen during endurance activities.[20]

Diets containing approximately 60% to 70% of ME are recommended for endurance exercise, and in times of extreme demand fat may supply up to 85% of ME, particularly in endurance sled dogs. Owners and trainers are best advised to introduce fats to the diet slowly, based on observations in the previous studies. A transition to higher-fat diets is best performed over approximately 8 to 12 weeks to allow for mitochondrial and metabolic adaptation.[30] A slow transition also reduces steatorrhea, which is a common acute adverse effect from feeding high-fat diets. Excess fat in the diet may require dietary increases in divalent cation nutrients (calcium, iron, zinc, copper, and manganese), which may chelate with free fatty acids, thereby reducing their bioavailability.[22] In addition, a word of caution is that addition of fat will dilute the protein, vitamin, and mineral content of the food, which creates a risk of insufficient intake of certain nutrients. In our opinion, if fat is added to a ration, this added fat should to exceed 20% to 25% of the overall ME of the diet for the typical athlete, except for rare instances of endurance sled dog racing where more might be required for a short period of time.

The ideal fat and carbohydrate composition in diets for racing greyhounds is highly debated,[31] with the most convincing evidence that dietary carbohydrate may play a role. Hill and colleagues[10,11] showed that greyhounds fed a diet with 43% ME as carbohydrates performed better than those on diets containing either 30% or 54% ME as carbohydrate when protein replaced carbohydrate. Additional studies showed that greyhounds fed 24% ME protein and 37% ME carbohydrate ran faster than those on a diet containing 37% ME protein and 24% ME carbohydrate when there was an isocaloric exchange of protein for carbohydrate.[32] These results, taken together with other protein intake data, suggest that diets with 24% ME from protein (60 g/1000 kcal) and between 30% to 50% ME from carbohydrate (75–125 g/1000 kcal) are most appropriate for racing greyhounds and other sprinting athletes. This nutrient composition, approximately 24% to 28% dry matter (DM) protein (65 g/1000 kcal), 12% to 14% DM fat (33 g/1000 kcal), and 45% to 50% DM carbohydrate (120 g/1000 kcal) would be found in many maintenance commercial kibbles. Many owners of sprinting, service, and intermediate athletic dogs that work for 30 minutes or less at a time are feeding high protein (>30% DM), fat (>20% DM) and less than 40% carbohydrate commercial kibbles. As their dogs do not work excessively hard for long periods of time, a commercial diet with a carbohydrate content of 40% to 50% DM similar to the one outlined as a maintenance commercial kibble previously, may be a better option. Endurance working dogs, such as field trial dogs, hunting dogs, long-distance sled dogs, and working herding dogs, are likely the ones that would benefit from commercial dry food of more than 30% DM protein and more than 20% DM fat, restricting carbohydrate content to 30% or lower.

PROTEIN REQUIREMENTS FOR THE CANINE ATHLETE

Protein requirements are really a requirement for essential amino acids in the diet. Most of the animal-based and plant-based protein sources provided in the commercial dog foods will provide essential and nonessential amino acids to the diet. Dogs synthesize nonessential amino acids through amination, deamination, and carboxylation reactions using carbon precursors and essential amino acids. Many of the studies on protein requirements use nitrogen balance studies (nitrogen in via diet vs nitrogen out in urine and feces) as the measure of adequacy. Nitrogen is a marker of protein, as protein is 16% nitrogen and by far the major source of nitrogen in the diet. However, most nitrogen balance studies do not take into account loss of lean body mass. There are multiple additional methods to evaluate dietary protein adequacy, each with its own merits and disadvantages. Dietary protein helps maintain muscle integrity and appropriate total protein, albumin, and hematocrit.[33] The hematocrit and serum albumin tend to decrease with training and racing, which appears to be a result of an overtraining syndrome[33,34] that may respond in part to increased protein intake. Based on studies involving sled dogs, one investigator has suggested that approximately 30% of daily metabolizable energy (70–80 g protein/1000 kcal) should come from highly digestible animal-based protein.[33] Four groups of sprint-racing sled dogs training in the field and on a treadmill were fed 4 different diets containing either 18% ME protein (48 g/1000 kcal), 24% ME protein (60 g/1000 kcal), 30% ME protein (75 g/1000 kcal), and 36% ME protein (90 g/1000 kcal). The dogs were examined 12 weeks after a transition from a 26% ME protein diet with similar ingredients. Complete blood counts, serum chemistries, VO_2 max (indirect calorimetry), and physical assessments were performed after 12 weeks of feeding each diet. Six of 8 dogs in the lowest-protein diet (18% ME) sustained musculoskeletal injuries and showed a 25% drop in VO_2 max. Dogs in the highest protein groups displayed a 10% increase in plasma volume, and there was a linear correlation between protein intake and hematocrit, hemoglobin, and total blood volume.[5] Querengaesser and colleagues[35] examined diets of approximately 28% to 34% ME protein (72 and 85 g/1000 kcal) and found no difference in the hematocrit decline over a 6-month training period, but the higher-protein group had elevated postexercise hematocrit, which could be just a reflection of dehydration. Exercise is thought to cause transient polycythemia followed by anemia and then a compensatory period of erythropoiesis; this latter phase may be a marker of adequate protein intake.[6] Protein quality and source also may be important. A study of mongrel dogs exercised 4 hours per day at 12 km/h compared unsupplemented soy protein versus fish meal–based and meat meal–based protein at approximately 35% ME. Dogs fed soybean meal had decreased hematocrit and increased red blood cell fragility after 3 weeks,[36] suggesting that soybean as the sole protein source may not be ideal. Endurance dogs should receive minimally 70 g/1000 kcal (approximately 26% of ME) of highly digestible animal-source or mixed animal/plant-based protein with no upper limit yet defined. The NRC suggests an adequate intake of 35% ME protein (90 g/1000 kcal) and 49% ME fat (59 g/1000 kcal) for endurance athletes.[6]

Sprinting dogs require less protein for exercise than endurance athletes. Hill and colleagues[32] performed studies suggesting that racing greyhounds perform better on lower-protein diets of 24% ME protein (63 g/1000 kcal) versus 43% ME protein (106 g/1000 kcal). Most racing greyhounds are provided 0.25 to 0.5 kg of meat mixed with dry commercial dog food daily to meet their energy requirements,[37] which provides an estimated 43% ME protein (106 g/1000 kcal), which is the same upper value used by Hill.[38] A recent study in detection dogs showed normal performance when fed a high-fat, low-protein diet containing 18% ME protein (45 g/1000 kcal) for 12 weeks. This amount of protein is lower than the Association of American Feed Control Officials (AAFCO) standards, but above the NRC requirements for protein, suggesting that low-protein diets may not be detrimental to all athletic endeavors; however, long-term feeding of low-protein diets and their overall effect on performance has not been evaluated.[39–43] Therefore, 24% ME protein (60 g/1000 kcal) is likely a reasonably adequate intake for sprinters and intermediate athletes not participating in long-duration endurance activities. Endurance athletes may require more dietary protein (closer to 30% ME or higher); however, definitive studies to elucidate the ideal amounts of protein in endurance athletes have yet to be performed.

BODY CONDITION AND EXERCISE

Body condition measures tend to be the great equalizer across all breeds of dog, allowing veterinarians and owners to evaluate the body of the athletic dog. The traditional body condition scoring methods use a 5-point or 9-point system. The 9-point system has been validated through comparison with dual x-ray absorptiometry analysis,[44] and is preferred by the authors. Most owners of performance dogs are aware of their animals' body condition scores and ideal competitive body weights. Typically performance dog owners maintain their dogs at a 4 to 5 of 9 body condition score (BCS). At these BCS values, ribs are easily palpable, there is an obvious abdominal tuck, a waist is visible from the side and top, and the dorsal aspect of the spinous processes can be felt. Greyhounds, field trial, hunting, and sprinting athletes may benefit from being maintained at a body condition score between 3 and 4 of 9. Dogs in this condition have ribs easily visualized in shorter-haired dogs, prominent spinous processes and wings of the ilea, but with ample paralumbar musculature that extends between the wings of the ilea so that the sacral spinous processes can be identified but do not protrude. Dogs in sprinting and intermediate activities (10–30 minutes) need to be lean to achieve ideal performance (**Fig. 1**), and restricted meal feeding during competition is common. In endurance activities in which speed is less important and in which there is a greater chance for loss of body condition during extended activity, a body condition score of 4 to 5 may be ideal to prevent severe weight loss.[45] On the other hand, service and some detection dogs observed in the field can run the gamut of body condition scores from 4 to 7; however, from a performance perspective, it would be ideal to keep most service dogs between 4 and 5 to prevent fatigue and joint-related problems associated with carrying excessive body weight.

FAT: BEYOND ENERGY

Many authors speculate that fatty acid chain length and saturation affect a variety of issues from inflammation to oxidative stress during exercise despite very little information regarding optimal dietary fat intakes for canine athletes.[46] Medium-chain triglycerides liberate 8-carbon to 12-carbon free fatty acids when digested, which are directly transported through absorption into the blood, bound to albumin, to the liver via the portal circulation. There are suggestions that medium-chain triglycerides in the form of coconut and palm oils are used more rapidly at the initiation of exercise, leading to sparing of glycogen.[47,48] One pilot study in athletic dogs showed limited utility.

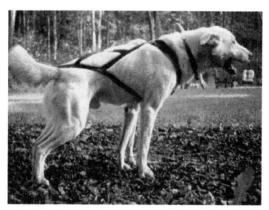

Fig. 1. Appropriate body condition for the canine athlete. Notice the rib cage showing just behind the elbow and the prominent musculature of the shoulder and hindlimb. This dog would be considered a 4 of 9 on the BCS chart. (*Courtesy of* Robert Downey, Sellersville, PA.)

Dietary increases in MCTs are not currently recommended as a strategy for working dogs.[49] The role of polyunsaturated fatty acids is described in greater detail with geriatric athlete nutrition, as the benefits on mobility and inflammation may be most pronounced in this population.

Fatty acid composition also could influence detection in scent-trained dogs and in many other performance animals that rely on scent, including foxhounds, hunting dogs, and service dogs. A small study showed that olfactory performance was diminished in dogs provided a diet rich in MCTs.[50] Another study using corn oil as a source of elevated polyunsaturated fatty acids (linoleic acid) demonstrated slightly improved find rates at detection thresholds in scent-trained Labradors.[39] The precise mechanism and magnitude of this effect has not yet been fully elucidated, but elevated polyunsaturated fatty acids may modestly improve performance in dogs that require olfactory acuity as part of their work.

CARBOHYDRATES: TIMING AND STRATEGY

The use of carbohydrate as a major dietary substrate is recommended in sprinting animals like greyhounds, ideally with approximately 40% to 50% of ME provided by highly digestible carbohydrates (100–125 g/1000 kcal). Endurance sled dogs require no more than 10% of ME as carbohydrates, and there is no definitive carbohydrate requirement in nonreproducing working dogs.[22,32] Carbohydrates also may be beneficial for sprinting and intermediate-distance athletes if muscle glycogen is depleted daily over the course of multiple-day events.[20,51,52] Studies in sled dogs demonstrated, for example, that postexercise supplementation with a maltodextrin supplement at 1.5 g/kg body weight within 30 minutes of exercise increased skeletal muscle glycogen within 4 to 24 hours.[51,52] Such strategic carbohydrate loading should be used only during competition to enhance glycogen repletion and should be done immediately after exercise and before any meals are provided to maximize absorption of the carbohydrate in a short period of time. If this type of supplementation was given daily during training, then the dog might use the increased carbohydrate for immediate energy preferentially rather than storing it as muscle glycogen. Therefore, postexercise carbohydrate repletion is recommended in dogs running between 5 minutes to 4 hours per day, particularly when expected to perform similarly the following day. The effectiveness of this strategy in endurance events is unknown and is not currently recommended by the authors.

DIETARY FIBER

Dietary fiber increases fecal bulk or moisture and is present in 2 forms: insoluble (nonfermentable) and soluble (fermentable). The increase in fecal volume during performance can lead to inappropriate defecation and increased fecal bulk, making the athlete slightly heavier. This is considered a negative attribute to fiber. On the other hand, during bouts of stress-diarrhea, insoluble fiber may affect gastrointestinal transit and reduce clinical signs of diarrhea. Soluble fibers may alter the large intestinal microflora, which produce short-chain fatty acids, some of which increase the absorptive surface of the large intestine through villous hypertrophy. Such properties have been used strategically in exercising canid athletes with stress-related diarrhea to ameliorate this condition. Several studies documented post-fiber production of volatile fatty acids, which promoted colonocyte regeneration and reduced recovery time from diarrhea.[53–55]

Many of the veterinary gastrointestinal therapeutic diets now contain small amounts of gums, soy fiber, fructooligosaccharides, other oligosaccharides, and mixed insoluble and soluble fiber sources (such as beet pulp) to improve fecal quality and intestinal absorptive surface area without increasing the overall fiber content of these diets too much. Commercial kibbles using whole grains, such as barley, oats, and sorghum, will naturally contain a mix of soluble and insoluble fiber and the true fiber content of many foods is unknown, as the crude fiber reported on the labels of commercial pet foods only represent the insoluble portion of fiber. The amount of soluble fiber in most performance and veterinary therapeutic foods is generally less than 2% of DM weight given that excess fermentation of this fiber source can decrease fecal quality by increasing the moisture content.[56] On the other hand, the addition of dietary psyllium husk powder in dogs can be helpful for resolving stress-diarrhea, which can be a common problem in working dogs. Psyllium husk fiber is a mucilage with water-binding properties and also acts like an insoluble fiber, providing a modest fermentation substrate for the microflora of the intestine. A starting dose of approximately 4 g fine psyllium powder (1 rounded teaspoon) daily has been recommended, with an upward titration to effect, not to exceed 16 g daily in a typical 20-kg to 30-kg canine athlete.[57]

ELECTROLYTES, MINERALS, AND VITAMINS IN THE WORKING CANINE

Minerals can be classified into major minerals and trace minerals. Deficiencies in major minerals have been observed in dogs fed nontraditional diets (meat-based without bone). Some athletic dogs, including racing greyhounds, are commonly fed all-meat diets. If raw or cooked meat-based diets are used, it is advisable that bones or bone meal be ground into the diet to improve the calcium and phosphorus balance. Calcium should be between 1.5 and 4.0 g/1000 kcal in most diets for adult athletic dogs (about 0.6%–1.2% DM), with similar amounts of phosphorus to maintain homeostasis for the structural integrity of bone, appropriate cellular signaling, and buffering capacity.[58] The calcium-to-phosphorus ratio is likely unimportant if adequate amounts of each are provided in the diet.[6] Deficiencies of the other major minerals, including sodium, potassium, and chloride have not been reported in adult working dogs, and therefore, the use of electrolyte supplements is not currently warranted when dogs are being sustained on commercial AAFCO-approved rations. The only studies that evaluated such mixtures showed either no beneficial effects or increased rates of diarrhea after activity.[59,60] Moreover, dogs cool primarily via panting, which is not associated with the same electrolyte losses as sweating in other species. The only dogs likely to benefit from electrolyte supplements may be dogs with protracted stress-diarrhea; veterinary diagnostics and other means of fluid therapy may be indicated in these cases.

Trace mineral intake will increase proportionally with the intake of commercial dog food, and will also increase, albeit to a lesser degree, when using raw or cooked meat to supplement commercial diets. If adding a fat source from animal or plant sources, the dilution of dietary vitamin and mineral intake will be even more egregious. Yet, to date, there are no reports of clinical deficiencies in copper, zinc, iron, manganese, iodine, or selenium in athletic canines being fed traditional commercial diets or commercial dog food and meat mixes. Currently it is unknown whether supplemental trace minerals are needed. Most exercising dogs have small to significant increases in caloric expenditure; as these animals will consume greater calories to maintain their body weight, they will also consume more of these minerals because the nutrient concentration of most diets is fixed.

Vitamins are classified as either fat-soluble or water-soluble. Water-soluble vitamins are typically included in the "B vitamin" family. Most of these vitamins are involved in cellular metabolism as intermediates or coenzymes within the citric acid cycle or as carriers and coenzymes for carbon transfer. An animal must be replete in these vitamins for normal energy metabolism. Most commercial dog foods and meats contain such vitamins well above the minimum requirement. Pet foods are typically supplemented with significant excesses of water-soluble vitamins to ensure adequate intake if there are any losses during production or storage, and these vitamins have large margins of safety.

The water-soluble vitamin C is synthesized in dogs through hepatic synthesis from glucose, unlike in humans and guinea pigs. However, dogs may not synthesize as much as other species.[61] The possibility for limitations in hepatic synthesis combined with observations that serum ascorbic acid concentrations decrease more than 50% after 190 minutes of sled racing have led to suggestions that supplementation may be beneficial.[33] Similar decreases in vitamin C were observed in unsupplemented greyhounds (1.8–2.8 mg/L).[62,63] Supplementation with 1 g ascorbic acid daily returns serum concentrations closer to what would be considered a normal baseline concentration (5–6 mg/L). However, similar supplementation in greyhounds for 4 weeks resulted in slower racing speeds by 0.3 km/h.[63] High doses of vitamin C also are associated with a pro-oxidant effect, which could be detrimental. Therefore, vitamin C supplementation cannot be recommended given the limited information available.

The fat-soluble vitamins (A, D, E, and K) have smaller margins of safety, and over-supplementation is the primary concern in performing athletes. Sufficient vitamin K is synthesized by bacterial flora in the gastrointestinal tract of normal dogs. Dietary vitamin A intake may be high if large quantities of organ meats are used in prepared or packaged meat-based diets, as liver tissue contains very high concentrations. Fortunately, dogs tend to be tolerant of high dietary vitamin A, although puppies and pregnant dogs have smaller safe upper limits.[64] Vitamin D also is found in organ meats, particularly liver, making a small amount of organ meat desirable if using meat as part of the diet (less than 15% as fed of total diet). Many commercial dog foods have at least twice the minimum requirement for cholecalciferol (vitamin D precursor), so with the increased energy consumption required by athletic dogs, the amount of cholecalciferol consumed should be adequate. Extremely high concentrations of vitamin D are associated with lethargy, gastrointestinal signs, and disorders in calcium homeostasis (parathyroid hormone, ionized calcium), with the most significant effects likely to occur during growth.

Vitamin E is sufficient in nearly all commercial pet foods, and most manufacturers add significantly more than the requirement, which makes vitamin E deficiency unlikely when feeding such diets. Deficiency has been observed in hunting dogs fed an all-meat diet, which led to retinal degeneration.[65] The effects of vitamin E have been examined extensively in endurance sled dogs. Low serum vitamin E levels were associated with an increased risk of failing to complete endurance sled dog races.[66] Additionally, serum vitamin E decreased after a single day of endurance activity in 2 separate studies.[33,67] Decreased serum vitamin E concentrations also have been observed in greyhounds racing 500 m.[68] Interestingly, compelling evidence for not supplementing high doses of vitamin E was provided by a study that showed that supplementing 100 to 1000 IU raised serum tocopherol concentrations, but that dogs receiving 1000 IU had slower racing times.[68,69]

Dietary composition is an important consideration. Diets high in polyunsaturated fatty acids (eg, fish-based sled dog diets) should contain higher amounts of vitamin E to prevent lipid peroxidation.[70] Diets high in selenium generally reduce vitamin E requirements, whereas those containing low amounts of selenium require more supplementation. However, tocopherol supplementation is generally not recommended in sporting dogs as long as they are being fed a complete and balanced dog food at their metabolic requirement. Dogs being fed nontraditional diets (primarily meats and fish) should consider vitamin E supplementation to prevent possible deficiency at a dose of 200 to 400 IU daily for a typical athletic dog of 40 to 80 pounds.

FEEDING STRATEGIES IN CANINE ATHLETES

Feeding patterns affect performance. The frequency and time of feeding can maximize metabolites that support increased activity and influence fecal volume, which affects competition. Sprinting dogs running for less than 20 minutes during a single bout of exercise benefit from modest feed restriction 24 hours before exercise (a decrease in total caloric intake of 20%–30%) to decrease fecal bulk. Some owners advocate small carbohydrate-rich meals before exercise to provide glucose as fuel for impending exercise, but there are few data to support this strategy in dogs.[71] However, sprinting and intermediate-distance athletes, particularly agility and field trial dogs, that perform multiple bouts of exercise in a day may benefit from immediate low-dose postexercise carbohydrate ingestion when they are expected to exercise again within 2 to 3 hours. If repetitive exercise is closer in frequency, feeding after exercise may not be recommended so as to avoid vomiting or regurgitation.[38] Postexercise glycogen repletion is advised for multiday events or trials, ideally administered within 30 minutes of the last exercise of the day.

Intermediate-distance athletes, which typically exercise once per day for 30 to 120 minutes, rely on both glycogen and fat for energy. Such animals should be fed diets moderate in protein and in carbohydrate (30% ME and 20% ME, respectively) and that are higher in fat (50% of ME). Fat will be used as a primary fuel at rest and fat oxidation will increase within 10 to 20 minutes of starting exercise to spare glycogen. This strategy of utilizing fat more readily available will allows dogs to run above 60% of VO_2 utilizing glycogen for more than 20 to 30 minutes. These athletes also benefit from postexercise carbohydrate supplementation to restore muscle glycogen concentrations, particularly during multiple-day events.[51,52] Provision of a single meal approximately 2 hours after exercise might be advantageous to promote continued lipolysis. Modest feed restriction (20%–30% of normal caloric intake) the day before competition decreases fecal bulk, helps prevent defecation during exercise, and promotes lipolysis.[11,16] Care should be taken to avoid feeding larger meals immediately after exercise, particularly in larger deep-chested breeds prone to gastric dilatation and volvulus. Dogs also should not be fed in the 8 hours before vigorous exercise to avoid a reduction in performance. Endurance athletes (ie, foxhounds and sled dogs) in heavy training tend to be fed 1 or 2 large meals daily, providing approximately 300 to 500 kcal/kg$^{0.75}$.[3,5,12,14] These meals should be approximately 30% ME protein (75 g/1000 kcal), 60% to 70% ME fat (>60 g/1000 kcal), and contain negligible carbohydrate, as described previously. However, data suggest that most mushers are feeding approximately 30% to 40% ME from protein (75–100 g/1000 kcal), 45% to 55% ME from fat (50–61 g/1000 kcal), and 10% to 20% from carbohydrate (25–50 g/1000 kcal).[72] Such rations are usually designed with 40% to 60% commercial dog food and the rest being high-fat meats so as to achieve the caloric density and digestibility needed for competitive racing and hunting. Search and rescue dogs, as well as foxhounds and pointing dogs that hunt or search for multiple hours over several days, may benefit from postexercise carbohydrate intake because they will rest for significant times (more than 8 hours) between exercises.

An entirely meat-based diet is not recommended by veterinary nutritionists or most veterinarians for endurance dogs because of the incomplete nature of such strategies, yet it is found as a common practice in some events and can be sustained for short periods of time without supplementation (5–10 days). Typically meats are provided raw, but most veterinary professionals recommend cooking the meat because cooking does not appear to decrease digestibility and might increase digestibility depending on the cooking process.[73] The extensive debate about the potential advantages and disadvantages of raw feeding are detailed elsewhere.[73]

All working dogs require more water than dogs at rest. Studies in sedentary dogs suggest that maintenance water requirements are between 0.6 and 1.0 mL/kcal ME.[6] However, dogs will continue to consume water even if the water concentration of the food is very high. The salt and protein content of the diet also influences drinking. As solutes (eg, Na and urea) increase, dogs adjust water intake. The amount of water required for exercise is dependent on the outside temperature, the ability to cool via evaporative means (panting), and the duration of the exercise (and therefore caloric expenditure). Some studies suggest that the timing of water administration after exercise is important.[74] For example, dogs in one study were offered water immediately after a run and drank to replace their losses; however, those dogs offered water 5 minutes after the run did not drink unless they were more than 0.5% dehydrated.[75] Racing greyhounds in training have been reported to increase daily water intake, resulting in an increase in plasma volume and a subsequent increase in blood volume. Dogs should be provided water immediately after intense exercise and routinely during training and feeding. Diets high in sodium are best avoided, as they may increase water intake and the severity of dehydration if it were to occur.

DIET IN THE GERIATRIC ATHLETE

Dogs display a slow deterioration of skeletal muscle mass known as sarcopenia with aging, a process that is likely similar to that documented in other species.[76] Dogs affected by peripheral neuropathies or chronic intervertebral disc disease also may display neurogenic atrophy, which can further exacerbate a decline in muscle condition score, and warrant rehabilitation or conditioning to help preserve lean body mass and to increase mobility. The VO_2 max decreases in geriatric dogs,[6] likely due to this reduction in muscle mass and efficiency. Dietary intervention is important in the aging athlete. Many "senior" dog foods restrict fat to reduce the caloric density and theoretically the propensity for obesity. Protein may be reduced in some diets due to a disproven theory that excess dietary protein accelerates the incidence and progression of renal disease.

However, it is likely that otherwise healthy senior performance animals should be fed diets high in caloric density and in protein. Older dogs also may have reductions in digestive capability, effectively decreasing the absorption of essential nutrients. Studies in young versus old dogs demonstrated that muscle protein turnover nearly doubles from 2.5 to approximately 5.0 g of protein per kilogram body weight daily in old dogs to maintain hepatic amino acid levels and skeletal muscle.[77] Unfortunately, evidence-based studies regarding the effects of diet in geriatric athletes are lacking. In the absence of definitive information, athletic senior dogs should receive approximately 5 g highly digestible protein per kg of body weight, or a diet containing more than 75 g/1000 kcal protein (26%–30% DM) and more than 35 g/1000 kcal fat (14%–16% DM). Normal adult dog or performance rations are the preferred choice when feeding older athletes, unless a "senior" diet conforms to the previously mentioned criteria or the senior athlete is experiencing weight gain because of reduced activity. For example, as some athletic dogs age, they may not be as active; therefore, caloric requirements decrease and a less energy-dense food may be desirable, which might be met by a commercial food with lower fat content (ie, 10%–14% DM fat). Currently there are few products on the market at more than 26% DM protein with fat content in the 10% to 14% DM range, although this may be ideal for some geriatric athletic dogs.

Geriatric animals are predisposed to arthritis, and performance athletes may suffer additional musculoskeletal pathology from repetitive strain injuries. Omega-3 fatty acids, specifically eicosapentaenoic acid (EPA) and docosahexaenoic acid (DHA), have received significant attention with respect to decreasing the clinical signs associated with osteoarthritis. Omega-3 fatty acids are polyunsaturated fatty acids. The most commonly studied include the 18-carbon alpha linolenic acid (ALA), the 20-carbon EPA, and the 22-carbon DHA. All unsaturated fatty acids are further characterized by the number of double bonds. The omega, or carbon "tail," position of the fatty acid contributes to nomenclature. Omega-3 fatty acids have a double bond in the third position from the methyl end; ALA contains 3 double bonds, EPA 5, and DHA 6. Dietary long-chain omega-3 fatty acids are incorporated in cellular membranes, and EPA serves as substrate for the COX and LOX enzymes. Omega-6 fatty acids are required in normal physiologic processes, but during inflammation are thought to contribute more to the formation of "proinflammatory" prostaglandins and leukotrienes, whereas omega-3 produces the less inflammatory 3-series prostanoids and 5-series leukotrienes.

The omega-3 fatty acids EPA and DHA have been studied in many clinically relevant conditions.[78] EPA and DHA are found in fish oils, although algal forms of DHA also exist. Dogs and humans have limited ability to convert ALA (found in flax seed and other oils) to EPA, and little to no conversion of ALA to DHA occurs. ALA-enriched diets must provide a high percentage (>7 times that needed of EPA/DHA) of fat as this precursor omega-3, because conversion to the longer-chain EPA and DHA is inefficient and at least 28 days are required to reach a steady state.[79] Any diet with elevated amounts of polyunsaturated fatty acids also requires increased amounts of vitamin E due to the increased lipid peroxidation from such supplementation.[80]

Diets containing elevated EPA and DHA have been recommended for degenerative joint disease,[81] with suggested daily doses of 230 to 370 mg combined EPA and DHA per body weight$^{0.75}$,[78] or roughly 2.5 to 4.0 g/1000 kcal in a diet for older dogs participating in short-distance performance activities. Common fish oil capsules contain about 300 mg of combined EPA and DHA. Therefore, a 25-kg dog requires 8 to 14 standard fish oil capsules daily to reach the recommended intake if the diet is low in these fatty acids, therefore dosing with teaspoon quantities of similar fish oil is recommended (2–3 teaspoons). EPA and DHA are thought to exert multiple functions in osteoarthritic joints. DHA may reduce intra-articular concentrations of proinflammatory cytokines, such as interleukin-1 and tumor necrosis factor, through eicosanoid modulation,[82] and there have been limited investigations of decreases in the matrix metalloproteinases that are involved in progressive cartilage degeneration following fish oil administration.[83]

Several clinical trials of fish oil–supplemented diets are available. One study of a commercial therapeutic joint diet with additional fish oil found that the greatest effect on scoring systems occurred with an estimated 7.5 g/1000 kcal of EPA and DHA.[84] Most commercial diets contain less than 0.5 g/1000 kcal for comparison. A multicenter study of a therapeutic joint diet, reported elsewhere to contain about 2.5 g of EPA and DHA per 1000 kcal, resulted in a decrease of carprofen dose from 4.4 mg/kg per day to 3.3 mg/kg per day in the treatment group, whereas the control group decreased from 4.2 mg/kg per day to 3.6 mg/kg per day over a 12-week period.[85] When fed for 90 days, the diet reportedly increased peak vertical force (PVF) by 5.6% in dogs versus

0.4% in dogs fed a control diet[86] and also improved osteoarthritis scoring.[87] A more recent investigation found that dogs fed fish oil (added to a base diet with an estimated 2.5 g EPA + DHA/1000 kcal total dietary intake) significantly increased PVF (+5.9%), decreased use of nonsteroidal anti-inflammatory drugs (NSAIDs), and increased quality-of-life scoring based on a visual analog scale when compared with a control group fed supplemental corn oil (estimated 0.04 g EPA + DHA/1000 kcal). Helsinki pain indices were reduced in both treatment and control groups, but the differences were not statistically significant because of a large standard deviation.[88]

There are significant differences between the nutrient profiles of diets purported to be suitable for the management of osteoarthritis.[81,89] Such diets are commonly recommended by practitioners, although over-the-counter fish-based diets also may contain high concentrations of omega-3 fatty acids. Liquid fish oil supplements are generally more cost-effective and pragmatic if fish oil is to be added to an unsupplemented diet. Fish oil will increase caloric intake if adjustments are not made to the base diet. Fish oil contains about 9 calories per gram, and a teaspoon of a fish oil product containing 1100 mg of combined EPA and DHA would add approximately 45 calories to the diet. At the current recommended dose of 2 to 3 tsp per day for a 25-kg dog, this would provide 90 to 135 additional kilocalories to the diet.

A variety of supplements are marketed for the management of osteoarthritis, some of which may be included in therapeutic diets labeled for such conditions. These include glucosamine, chondroitin, methylsulfonylmethane, avocado and soybean unsaponifiables, fatty acid products, green-lipped mussel, and turmeric. A recent meta-analysis of canine supplements for this purpose documented clear benefits for omega-3 fatty acids but only limited evidence for all supplements examined.[90] The most common joint supplements are products designed as chondroprotectants. Proteoglycans are thought to be critical in maintaining the features of cartilage, such as flexibility and elasticity, and are stabilized with long chains of hyaluronic acid. Glucosamine is a precursor to hyaluronic acid and other glycosaminoglycans. Chondroitin sulfate is also a precursor to major glycosaminoglycans, which in turn are complexed to proteins like aggrecan, to provide proteoglycans. These compounds are commonly used in humans and in animals, although efficacy has been significantly questioned in human meta-analyses.[91]

Both radiolabeled glucosamine and chondroitin are absorbed orally in dogs when administered as a radiolabeled supplement.[92] A double-blinded positive-controlled trial of a product dosed at 475 mg glucosamine HCl, 350 mg chondroitin sulfate, 50 mg N-acetyl-D-glucosamine, 50 mg ascorbic acid, and 30 mg Zn sulfate per about 20 kg of body weight found that subjective osteoarthritis scores were improved at 70 days with this product as compared with 42 days with carprofen (4 mg/kg/d for 7 days, 2 mg/kg/d for maintenance). Improvements were not significantly different between groups at day 70.[93] A shorter study compared a different glucosamine and chondroitin product to meloxicam and to carprofen, but only for 60 days, and found improvements only with the NSAIDs as measured by ground reaction forces and subjective scores.[94] Studies of other supplements included in therapeutic diets, such as green-lipped mussel containing omega-3 fatty acids, minerals, and other compounds, found that some owners perceive huge improvements in osteoarthritis even when dogs are given placebo.[95] Further research is necessary before definitive recommendations can be made on the efficacy of chondroprotectants. In the interim, if glucosamine and chondroitin are included in the medical management of osteoarthritis in the canine athlete, the compounds should likely be dosed at about 25 mg/kg and 15 mg/kg, respectively, and owners should be cautioned that improvements may not be evident for several months. The glucosamine and chondroitin concentrations in commercial pet foods are generally lower than those available in supplement form, and joint diets often do not contain appreciably more than normal commercial pet foods.[89]

Sporadic studies have examined evidence for the inclusion of supplements in the diets for geriatric pets. There is some evidence that acetyl-l-carnitine (27.5 mg/kg) and alpha-lipoic acid (11 mg/kg) improve cognitive performance in older animals, which could have applications for the canine athlete.[96] Carnitine is required for the transport of fatty acids across the mitochondrial membrane, and alpha-lipoic acid is an essential component of the pyruvate dehydrogenase complex, which converts pyruvate to acetyl-CoA. As a result, both are essential for normal cellular metabolism. Some over-the-counter supplements marketed for osteoarthritis contain herbal products. Uncontrolled trials of Boswellia resin (frankincense) in dogs have been reported,[97] which expand on some limited, but favorable, human trials. Curcumin, an extract from the spice turmeric, is another frequent inclusion in canine supplements because of its reported nuclear factor–κB inhibition, but this has been studied only in humans.[98] Additional information is required about these and other dietary supplements before determining their safety and efficacy.

DIETS FOR FUTURE CANINE ATHLETES: NUTRITIONAL CONSIDERATIONS DURING GROWTH

Future athletic performance is influenced by environmental and nutritional factors during growth. Nutrient flexibility will be reduced during growth, making nutrient balance more critical than in adults. Calcium homeostasis is of particular concern, as unbalanced or all-meat diets will predispose puppies to osteopenia and pathologic fractures.[99,100] Puppies generally have higher protein, essential fatty acid, and mineral requirements on a caloric basis.[70,101,102] Modulation of certain nutrients could produce benefits during early behavioral or performance training. DHA, for example, has been shown to improve a variety of cognitive and psychomotor parameters in puppies up to 1 year of age.[103] The diet with the greatest effect contained an estimated 1.25 g EPA and DHA per 1000 kcal (500 mg DHA/1000 kcal), but was also supplemented with additional vitamin E, taurine, choline, and L-carnitine, all of which could affect learning and memory.

Diets for large-breed puppies should be selected to control calcium and calorie intake. Excess calcium intake in large-breed puppies, such as Great Danes, has been associated with alterations in endochondral ossification, delayed skeletal maturation, and decreased osteoclastic activity.[104] Passive diffusion of calcium is increased in growing puppies, creating a linear absorption not observed in adults.[105] Excess vitamin D also may be problematic because of the increased concentration of 24,25-hydroxyvitamin D, which may adversely affect skeletal maturation. Diets for large-breed puppies should contain 3.0 to 4.5 g/1000 kcal calcium to prevent nutritional induction of skeletal abnormalities.[70]

Maintenance of lean body weight is critical during growth. Most puppies consume the same daily caloric intake at 4 months of age as they do when fully grown at 2 years old. As a result, if the weight of the same-gendered parent is known, this value can be used to approximate daily energy requirements after 4 months using the following equation: $130 \times$ (parental body weight in kg)$^{0.75}$ kcal/day. This equation approximates the calculated values for complex equations given by the NRC and other sources. Ad libitum feeding and overnutrition are associated with a greater incidence of osteochondrosis lesions,[106] skeletal abnormalities,[107] and hip dysplasia,[108] presumably because of the structural effects of excess weight[107] combined with other factors.

The provision of diets labeled for growth should be sufficient to prevent nutritionally induced developmental orthopedic disease. However, large-breed dogs may benefit from large-breed formulations, which generally contain less than 4 g calcium/1000 kcal and allow for modest energy restriction to maintain appropriate body condition. Some all-life-stages foods may contain excess calcium for such dogs, as they are formulated to provide adequacy for pregnancy and lactation. There is no evidence that elevated protein causes skeletal abnormalities or developmental orthopedic disease. Therefore, the practice of feeding adult pet foods to growing puppies of any breed is unfounded. Such foods would be expected to be deficient in one or more nutrients required for growth.

The concept of conditioning and training a dog during dynamic growth is equally important in puppies. Rigorous conditioning programs are not advised because of potential growth plate damage. All training and conditioning activities should be low intensity and low impact to prevent such damage during dynamic growth in puppies younger than 6 months of age. Training should be gradually increased over time and rigorous training activities are not advised until skeletal maturity, which is often between 9 and 12 months of age for the average performance dog. Therefore "pushing" young dogs may lead to musculoskeletal injury with long-term detrimental consequences.

SUMMARY

Canine endurance athletes benefit from nutritional strategies tailored to their high rates of aerobic fat metabolism. The caloric expenditure of most exercise is best predicted by assessing the distance traveled rather than the speed or intensity of the activity. Sprinting athletes, such as racing greyhounds, agility dogs, and other high-intensity short-duration activities have modest increases in daily energy expenditure (<25%) and benefit from a diet moderate in carbohydrate, protein, and in fat, similar to most maintenance pet foods. Endurance, prolonged hunting, field trial, working herding, or long-distance activities require larger increases in daily food intake and often need supplemental fat to meet energy demands of exercise. Appropriate diets for such dogs are moderate in protein (>75 g/1000 kcal) and high in fat (>60 g/1000 kcal). Post-exercise carbohydrate supplementation may replenish glycogen stores in dogs competing for several straight days, and water should always be offered immediately after exercise to prevent dehydration. Aging athletes require increases in dietary protein to preserve lean body mass and benefit from elevations in dietary omega-3 fatty acids. Growing large-breed puppies with performance potential should be maintained in ideal body condition during growth by feeding a diet with appropriate amounts of calcium. Service dogs typically live within the lifestyle of those that they serve and may have nutritional needs similar to normal active dogs; however, they should be watched for unnecessary weight gain that may hinder their ability to work as efficiently. Additional research is needed for activity-specific nutritional requirements to better understand the role of performance nutrition in the diverse sports/service work in which dogs and owners participate.

REFERENCES

1. Beitz DC. Comparative digestive physiology of dogs and cats. In: National Research Council (NRC), editor. Nutrient requirements of dogs and cats. Washington, DC: National Academy Press; 2006. p. 5–21.
2. Kienzle E. Energy. In: National Research Council (NRC), editor. Nutrient requirements of dogs and cats. Washington, DC: National Academy Press; 2006. p. 29–48.

3. Musch TL, Haidet GC, Ordway GA, et al. Dynamic exercise training in fox-hounds. I. Oxygen consumption and hemodynamic responses. J Appl Physiol 1985;59:183–9.

4. Ordway GA, Floyd DL, Longhurst JC, et al. Oxygen consumption and hemodynamic responses during graded treadmill exercise in the dog. J Appl Physiol 1984;57:601–7.

5. Reynolds AJ, Reinhart GA, Carey DP, et al. Effect of protein intake during training on biochemical and performance variables in sled dogs. Am J Vet Res 1999;60:789–95.

6. Hill RC. Physical activity and environment. In: National Research Council (NRC), editor. Nutrient requirements of dogs and cats. Washington, DC: National Academy Press; 2006. p. 258–312.

7. Taylor CR, Caldwell SL, Rowntree VJ. Running up and down hills: some consequences of size. Science 1972;178:1096–7.

8. Schmidt-Nielsen J. Scaling: why is animal size so important. Cambridge (United Kingdom): Cambridge University Press; 1984.

9. Taylor RJ. The work output of sledge dogs. J Physiol 1957;137:210–7.

10. Hill RC, Bloomberg MS, Legrand-Defretin V, et al. Maintenance energy requirements and the effects of diet on performance in racing greyhounds. Am J Vet Res 2000;61:1566–73.

11. Hill RC, Lewis DD, Scott KC, et al. Mild food restriction increases the speed of racing greyhounds. J Vet Intern Med 1999;13:281.

12. Decombaz J, Jambon M, Pigueet C, et al. Energy intake and expenditure of sled dogs during the Alpirod race. In: Grandjean D, Vanek J, editors. Proceedings 2nd Annual Sled Dog Veterinary Medical Association Symposium. 1995. p. 113–8.

13. Orr NW. The feeding of sledge dogs on Antarctic expeditions. J Nutr 1966;20: 1–12.

14. Hinchcliff KW, Reinhart GA, Burr JR, et al. Metabolizable energy intake and sustained energy expenditure of Alaskan sled dogs during heavy exertion in the cold. Am J Vet Res 1997;58:1457–62.

15. Ahlstrom O, Redman P, Speakman J. Energy expenditure and water turnover in hunting dogs in winter conditions. Br J Nutr 2011;106:S158–61.

16. Toll PW, Gillette RL. The canine athlete. In: Hand MS, Thatcher CD, Remillard RL, et al, editors. Small animal clinical nutrition. 5th edition. Marceline (MO): Walsworth Publishing; 2010. p. 323–57.

17. Wagner JA, Horvath SM, Dahms TE. Cardiovascular, respiratory and metabolic adjustments to exercise. J Appl Phys 1977;42:403–7.

18. Granjean D. Nutrition for sled dogs. In: Dee JF, Bloomberg MS, Taylor RA, editors. Canine sports medicine and surgery. Philadelphia: WB Saunders Co; 1998. p. 336–47.

19. Reynolds AJ, Fuhrer L, Dunlap HL, et al. Effect of diet and training on muscle glycogen storage and utilization in sled dogs. J Appl Physiol 1995;79:1601–7.

20. McKenzie EC, Hinchcliff KW, Valberg SJ, et al. Assessment of alterations in triglyceride and glycogen concentrations in muscle tissue of Alaskan sled dogs during repetitive prolonged exercise. Am J Vet Res 2008;69:1097–103.

21. McClelland G, Zwingelstein G, Taylor CR, et al. Increased capacity for circulatory fatty acid transport in a highly aerobic mammal. Am J Physiol 1994;266: R1280–6.

22. Reinhart GA. Nutrition for sporting dogs. In: Dee JF, Bloomberg MS, Taylor RA, editors. Canine sports medicine and surgery. Philadelphia: WB Saunders Co; 1998. p. 348–56.

23. Gunn HM. Differences in the histochemical properties of skeletal muscles of different breeds of horses and dogs. J Anat 1978;127:615–34.

24. Maxwell LC, Barclay JK, Mohrman DE, et al. Physiological characteristics of skeletal muscles of dogs and cats. Am J Physiol 1977;233:C14–8.

25. Downey RL, Kronfeld DS, Banta CA. Diet of beagles affects stamina. J Am Anim Hosp Assoc 1980;16:273–7.

26. Hargreaves M, Costill DL, Coggan A, et al. Effect of carbohydrate feedings on muscle glycogen utilization and exercise performance. Med Sci Sports Exerc 1984;16:219–22.

27. Wakshlag JJ, Cooper BJ, Wakshlag RR, et al. Biochemical evaluation of mitochondrial respiratory chain enzymes in canine skeletal muscle. Am J Vet Res 2004;65:480–4.

28. Kronfeld DS, Hammel EP, Ramberg CF, et al. Hematological and metabolic responses to training in racing sled dogs fed diets containing medium, low and zero carbohydrate. Am J Clin Nutr 1977;30:419–30.

29. Hammel EP, Kronfeld DS, Ganjam VK, et al. Metabolic responses to exhaustive exercise in racing sled dogs fed diets containing medium, low or zero carbohydrate. Am J Clin Nutr 1977;30:409–18.

30. Reynolds AJ, Fuhrer L, Dunlap HL, et al. Lipid metabolite responses to diet and training in sled dogs. J Nutr 1994;124:2754S–9S.

31. Toll PW, Pieschl RL, Hand MS. The effect of dietary fat and carbohydrate on sprint performance in racing greyhound dogs. Proceedings of the 8th International Racing Greyhound Symposium, North American Veterinary Conference. Orlando (FL):1992. p. 1–3.

32. Hill RC, Lewis DD, Scott KC, et al. The effects of increased protein and decreased carbohydrate in the diet on performance and body composition in racing greyhounds. Am J Vet Res 2001;62:440–7.

33. Kronfeld DS, Adkins TO, Downey RL. Nutrition, anaerobic and aerobic exercise and stress. In: Burger IH, Rivers JP, editors. Cambridge (UK): Cambridge University Press; Nutrition of dog and cat: Waltham Symposium. 1989. p. 133–45.

34. Wakshlag JJ, Stokol T, Geske SM, et al. Evaluation of exercise-induced changes in concentrations of C-reactive protein and serum biochemical values in sled dogs completing a long-distance endurance race. Am J Vet Res 2010;71:1207–13.

35. Querengaesser A, Iben C, Leibetseder J. Blood changes during training and racing in sled dogs. J Nutr 1994;124:2760S–4S.

36. Yamada TM, Tohori T, Ashida T, et al. Comparison of effects of vegetable protein diet and animal protein diet on the initiation of anemia during vigorous physical training in dogs and rats. J Nutr Sci Vitaminol (Tokyo) 1987;33:129–49.

37. Kohnke JR. Nutrition in the racing greyhound. In: Dee JF, Bloomberg MS, Taylor RA, editors. Canine sports medicine and surgery. Philadelphia: WB Saunders Co; 1998. p. 328–36.

38. Hill RC. The nutritional requirements of exercising dogs. J Nutr 1998;128: S2686–90.

39. Angle TC, Wakshlag JJ, Gillette RS, et al. The effects of exercise and diet on olfaction in detection dogs. J Nutr Sci, in press.

40. Wakshlag JJ, Kallfelz FA, Barr SC, et al. Effects of exercise on canine skeletal muscle proteolysis: an investigation of the ubiquitin proteasome pathway and other metabolic markers. Vet Ther 2002;3:215–25.

41. Wasserman DH, Williams PE, Lacy DB, et al. Importance of intrahepatic mechanisms to gluconeogenesis from alanine during exercise and recovery. Am J Physiol 1988;254:E518–25.

42. Wasserman DH, Spalding JA, Lacy DB, et al. Glucagon is a primary controller of hepatic glycogenolysis and gluconeogenesis during muscular work. Am J Physiol 1989;257:E108–17.
43. Wasserman DH, Geer RJ, Williams PE, et al. Interaction of gut and liver in nitrogen metabolism during exercise. Metabolism 1991;40:307–14.
44. Laflamme DP. Development and validation of a body condition score system for dogs. Can Pract 1997;22:10–5.
45. Hinchcliff KW, Shaw LC, Vukich NS, et al. Effect of distance traveled and speed of racing on body weight and serum enzyme activity of sled dogs competing in a long distance race. J Am Vet Med Assoc 1998;213:639–44.
46. Bauer JE. Facilitative and functional fats in diets of cats and dogs. J Am Vet Med Assoc 2006;229:680–4.
47. Jeukendrup AE, Aldred S. Fat supplementation, health, and endurance performance. Nutrition 2004;20:678–88.
48. Hawley JA. Effect of increased fat availability on metabolism and exercise capacity. Med Sci Sports Exerc 2002;34:1485–91.
49. Reynolds AJ. The role of fat in the formulation of performance rations: focus on fat sources. In: Hayek MG, Lepine AJ, Sunvold GD, editors. Recent advances in canine and feline nutrition. vol. II. Wilmington (OH): Orange Frazer Press; 1998. p. 277–81.
50. Altom EK, Davenport GM, Myers LJ, et al. Effect of dietary fat source and exercise on odorant-detecting ability of canine athletes. Res Vet Sci 2003;75:149–55.
51. Reynolds AJ, Carey DP, Reinhart GA, et al. Effect of post-exercise carbohydrate supplementation on muscle glycogen repletion in trained sled dogs. Am J Vet Res 1997;58:1252–6.
52. Wakshlag JJ, Sneddon KA, Otis AM, et al. Effects of post-exercise supplements on glycogen repletion in skeletal muscle. Vet Ther 2002;3:226–34.
53. Gagné JW, Wakshlag JJ, Simpson KW, et al. Effects of a synbiotic on fecal quality, short-chain fatty acid concentrations, and the microbiome of healthy racing sled dogs. BMC Vet Res 2013;9:246.
54. Wakshlag JJ, Struble AM, Simpson KW, et al. Negative fecal characteristics are associated with pH and fecal flora alterations during dietary change in dogs. BMC Vet Res 2010;9:278–83.
55. Whelan K, Schneider SM. Mechanisms, prevention, and management of diarrhea in enteral nutrition. Curr Opin Gastroenterol 2011;27:152–9.
56. Beloshapka AN, Wolff AK, Swanson KS. Effects of feeding polydextrose on faecal characteristics, microbiota and fermentative end products in healthy adult dogs. Br J Nutr 2011;16:1–7.
57. Lieb MS. Treatment of chronic idiopathic large bowel diarrhea in dogs with a highly digestible diet and soluble fiber: a retrospective review of 37 cases. J Vet Intern Med 2000;14:27–32.
58. Kallfetz FA. Minerals. In: National Research Council (NRC), editor. Nutrient requirements of dogs and cats. Washington, DC: National Academy Press; 2006. p. 145–92.
59. Mazin RM, Fordyce HH, Otto CM. Electrolyte replacement in urban search and rescue dogs: a field study. Vet Ther 2001;2:140–7.
60. Young DR, Schafer NS, Price R. Effect of nutrient supplements during work on performance. J Appl Physiol 1960;15:1022–6.
61. Chatterjee IB, Majumder BK, Nandi BK, et al. Synthesis and some major functions of vitamin C in animals. Ann N Y Acad Sci 1975;258:24–47.

62. Scott KC, Hill RC, Lewis DD, et al. Serum ascorbic acid concentrations in previously unsupplemented greyhounds after administration of a single dose of ascorbic acid intravenously or per os. J Anim Physiol Anim Nutr 2002;86:222–8.

63. Marshall RJ, Scott KC, Hill RC, et al. Supplemental vitamin C appears to slow racing greyhounds. J Nutr 2002;132:1616S–21S.

64. Morris P, Salt C, Raila J, et al. The effects of feeding vitamin A to puppies up to 52 weeks of age. Waltham International Science Symposium: pet nutrition – art or science? Cambridge (UK); 2011. p. 52.

65. Davidson MG, Geoly FJ, Gilger BC, et al. Retinal degeneration associated with vitamin E deficiency in hunting dogs. J Am Vet Med Assoc 1998;213:645–51.

66. Piercy RJ, Hinchcliff KW, Morely PS, et al. Association between vitamin E and enhanced athletic performance in sled dogs. Med Sci Sports Exerc 2001;33: 826–33.

67. Piercy RJ, Hinchcliff KW, Morely PS, et al. Vitamin E and exertional rhabdomyolysis during endurance sled dog racing. Neuromuscul Disord 2001;11: 278–86.

68. Scott KC, Hill RC, Lewis DD, et al. Effect of oral alpha tocopherol acetate supplementation on vitamin E concentrations in greyhounds before and after a race. Am J Vet Res 2001;62:1118–20.

69. Hill RC, Armstrong D, Browne RW, et al. Chronic administration of high doses of vitamin E appears to slow racing greyhounds. FASEB J 15:A990.

70. Morris JG, Vitamins National Research Council (NRC). Nutrient requirements of dogs and cats. Washington, DC: National Academy Press; 2006. p. 193–245.

71. Hawley JA, Schabort EJ, Noakes TD, et al. Carbohydrate-loading and exercise performance. An update. Sports Med 1997;24:73–81.

72. Loftus JP, Molly Yazwinski M, Millizio JG, et al. Energy requirements for racing endurance sled dogs. J Nutr Sci, in press.

73. Freeman LM, Chandler ML, Hamper BA, et al. Current knowledge about the risks and benefits or raw meat diets for dogs and cats. J Am Vet Med Assoc 2013;243(11):1549–58.

74. Wakshlag JJ, Sneddon KA, Reynolds AJ. Biochemical and metabolic changes due to exercise in sprint-racing sled dogs: implications for postexercise carbohydrate supplements and hydration management. Vet Ther 2004;5:52–9.

75. O'Conner WJ. Drinking by dogs during and after running. J Physiol 1975;250: 247–59.

76. Freeman LM. Cachexia and sarcopenia: emerging syndromes of importance in dogs and cats. J Vet Intern Med 2012;26:3–17.

77. Wannemacher RW, McCoy JR. Determination of optimal dietary protein requirements in young and old dogs. J Nutr 1966;88:66–74.

78. Bauer JE. Therapeutic use of fish oils in companion animals. J Am Vet Med Assoc 2011;239:1441–51.

79. Dunbar BL, Bigley KE, Bauer JE. Early and sustained enrichment of serum n-3 long chain polyunsaturated fatty acids in dogs fed a flaxseed supplemented diet. Lipids 2010;45:1–10.

80. Walters JM, Hackett TB, Ogilvie GK, et al. Polyunsaturated fatty acid dietary supplementation induces lipid peroxidation in normal dogs. Vet Med Int 2010; 2010:619083.

81. Perea S. Nutritional management of osteoarthritis. Compendium 2012;35:E1–3.

82. Zainal Z, Longman AJ, Hurst S, et al. Relative efficacies of omega-3 polyunsaturated fatty acids in reducing expression of key proteins in a model system for studying osteoarthritis. Osteoarthr Cartil 2009;17:896–905.

83. Hansen RA, Harris MA, Pluhar GE, et al. Fish oil decreases matrix metalloproteinases in knee synovia of dogs with inflammatory joint disease. J Nutr Biochem 2008;19:101–8.

84. Fritsch D, Allen TA, Dodd CE, et al. Dose-titration effects of fish oil in osteoarthritic dogs. J Vet Intern Med 2010;24:1020–6.

85. Fritsch DA, Allen TA, Dodd CE, et al. A multicenter study of the effect of dietary supplementation with fish oil omega-3 fatty acids on carprofen dosage in dogs with osteoarthritis. J Am Vet Med Assoc 2010;236:535–9.

86. Roush JK, Cross AR, Renberg WC, et al. Evaluation of the effects of dietary supplementation with fish oil omega-3 fatty acids on weight bearing in dogs with osteoarthritis. J Am Vet Med Assoc 2010;236:67–73.

87. Roush JK, Dodd CE, Fritsch DA, et al. Multicenter veterinary practice assessment of the effects of omega-3 fatty acids on osteoarthritis in dogs. J Am Vet Med Assoc 2010;236:59–66.

88. Hielm-Bjorkman A, Roine J, Elo K, et al. An un-commissioned randomized, placebo-controlled double-blind study to test the effect of deep sea fish oil as a pain reliever for dogs suffering from canine OA. BMC Vet Res 2012;8:157–69.

89. Shmalberg J. Canine rehabilitative and performance nutrition. Proceedings of the North American Veterinary Conference. Orlando (FL): 2013. p. 68–70.

90. Vandeweerd JM, Coisnon C, Clegg P, et al. Systematic review of efficacy of nutraceuticals to alleviate clinical signs of osteoarthritis. J Vet Intern Med 2012;26: 448–56.

91. Wandel S, Juni P, Tendal B, et al. Effects of glucosamine, chondroitin, or placebo in patients with osteoarthritis of the hip or knee: network meta-analysis. BMJ 2010;341:4675.

92. Adebowale A, Du J, Liang Z, et al. The bioavailability and pharmacokinetics of glucosamine hydrochloride and low molecular weight chondroitin sulfate after sing and multiple doses to beagle dogs. Biopharm Drug Dispos 2002;23(6): 217–25.

93. McCarthy G, O'Donovan J, Jones B, et al. Randomised double-blind, positive-controlled trial to assess the efficacy of glucosamine/chondroitin sulfate for the treatment of dogs with osteoarthritis. Vet J 2007;174:54–61.

94. Moreau M, Dupuis J, Bonneau NH, et al. Clinical evaluation of a nutraceutical, carprofen and meloxicam for the treatment of dogs with osteoarthritis. Vet Rec 2003;152:323–9.

95. Pollard B, Guilford WG, Ankenbauer-Perkins KL, et al. Clinical efficacy and tolerance of an extract of green-lipped mussel (*Perna canaliculus*) in dogs presumptively diagnosed with degenerative joint disease. N Z Vet J 2006; 54:114–8.

96. Milgram NW, Araujo JA, Hagen TM, et al. Acetyl-l-carnitine and alpha-lipoic acid supplementation of aged beagle dogs improves learning in two landmark discrimination tests. FASEB J 2007;21:3756–62.

97. Reichling J, Schmokel H, Fitzi J, et al. Dietary support with Boswellia resin in canine inflammatory joint and spinal disease. Schweiz Arch Tierheilkd 2004; 16:71–9.

98. Chandran B, Goel A. A randomized, pilot study to assess the efficacy and safety of curcumin in patients with active rheumatoid arthritis. Phytother Res 2012;26: 1719–25.

99. Taylor MB, Geiger DA, Saker KE, et al. Diffuse osteopenia and myelopathy in a puppy fed a diet composed of an organic premix and raw ground beef. J Am Vet Med Assoc 2009;234:1041–8.

100. Malik R, Laing C, Davis PE, et al. Rickets in a litter of racing greyhounds. J Small Anim Pract 1997;38:109–14.
101. Rogers O. Protein and amino acids. In: National Research Council (NRC), editor. Nutrient requirements of dogs and cats. Washington, DC: National Academy Press; 2006. p. 111–45.
102. Bauer JE. Fats and fatty acids. In: National Research Council (NRC), editor. Nutrient requirements of dogs and cats. Washington, DC: National Academy Press; 2006. p. 81–110.
103. Zicker SC, Jewell DE, Yamka RM, et al. Evaluation of cognitive learning, memory, psychomotor, immunologic, and retinal functions in healthy puppies fed foods fortified with docosahexaneoic acid-rich fish oil from 8 to 52 weeks of age. J Am Vet Med Assoc 2012;241:583–94.
104. Hazelwinkel HA, Goedegebuure SA, Poulos PW, et al. Influences of chronic calcium excess on the skeletal development of growing Great Danes. J Am Anim Hosp Assoc 1985;21:337–91.
105. Tryfonidou MA, Van den Broek J, Van den Brom WE, et al. Intestinal calcium absorption in growing dogs is influenced by calcium intake and age but not by growth rate. J Nutr 2002;132:3363–8.
106. Lavelle RB. The effect of overfeeding of a balanced complete commercial diet to a young group of Great Danes. In: Burger IH, Rivers JP, editors. Nutrition of the dog and cat. Cambridge (UK): Cambrdige Univ Press; 1989. p. 303–15.
107. Meyer H, Zentek J. Energy requirements of growing Great Danes. J Nutr 1991; 121:S35–6.
108. Kealy RD, Olsson SE, Monti KL, et al. Effects of limited food consumption on the incidence of hip dysplasia in growing dogs. J Am Vet Med Assoc 1992;201: 857–63.

Nutrition of Aging Dogs

Jennifer A. Larsen, DVM, PhD[a],*, Amy Farcas, DVM, MS[b]

KEYWORDS

- Aging • Geriatric • Canine • Senior • Diet • Nutrition

KEY POINTS

- There are increasing numbers of geriatric dogs in the United States; this population is characterized by normal aging processes as well as an increased frequency of age-related diseases, including osteoarthritis, cognitive dysfunction, chronic kidney disease, and neoplasia.
- Although there are potentially important physiologic effects of aging on the digestive process, most studies report no differences in nutrient absorption when comparing young adult with geriatric dogs.
- Nutritional factors that may be important in the management of aged dogs include energy density of the diet and intake of protein, phosphorus, and sodium as well as specific nutrients and nutraceuticals that are of interest for addressing age-related disease.

INTRODUCTION
Relevance

Aged dogs are a common population seen by clinicians, and both the proportion of older dogs and the age seem to be increasing. It is estimated that more than 43 million US households owned a dog in 2011.[1] A 2012 e-mail survey of 50,347 respondents revealed that 33.2% of dogs were 6 to 10 years of age and 14.7% were older than 11 years; over the prior 5 years, this represents an increase of 9.1% in the number of dogs older than 6 years.[1] These increases are modest compared with slightly older data reporting 30% of dogs were aged 7 to 11 years and 9% were 12 to 15 years old.[2] In 2012, the average life span of one population of dogs was 11 years, which represents an increase of 0.5 years over the prior 10 years.[3,4]

When Are Dogs Considered Seniors?

The age of transition of dogs from adult to senior or geriatric is variable and subjective. One study reported that according to the labels of 37 commercial foods marketed for senior dogs, dogs were considered to be senior starting at a range of 5 to more than 8 years of age, whereas pet owners considered this range to be 5 to more than

---

[a] VM: Molecular Biosciences, School of Veterinary Medicine, University of California, Davis, One Shields Avenue, Davis, CA 95616, USA; [b] Department of Clinical Studies, School of Veterinary Medicine, University of Pennsylvania, Philadelphia, PA 19104, USA
* Corresponding author.
E-mail address: jalarsen@vmth.ucdavis.edu

Vet Clin Small Anim 44 (2014) 741–759
http://dx.doi.org/10.1016/j.cvsm.2014.03.003
0195-5616/14/$ – see front matter © 2014 Elsevier Inc. All rights reserved.

10 years of age.[5] Dogs vary widely in expected life span and body size dependent partly on breed, and there is a well-recognized negative correlation between breed size and life expectancy.[6,7] The transition age may be best considered relative to the individual's genetic makeup and phenotype because different rates of aging can be apparent among different dogs. The Senior Care Guidelines Task Force of the American Animal Hospital Association suggests that pets are considered seniors when in the last 25% of their predicted life span based on species and breed.[8] It is important to note that life stages are defined by the age of populations rather than individuals. Regardless, despite the arbitrary nature of the age at which dogs are considered to be seniors, there are documented biologic effects of advancing age as well as increasing incidence of the onset and/or progression of various chronic diseases; many of these issues may be influenced through various nutritional strategies.[9]

ASSESSMENT

Regular, comprehensive assessment of physical, lifestyle, and nutritional factors is warranted for all senior dogs (**Boxes 1** and **2**). There are 2 aspects to the approach to care of this population of dogs. The first involves screening for and addressing/accommodating physiologic changes caused by the normal aging of healthy older dogs; this population is clinically well and has no significant clinicopathologic findings on assessment. The second aspect is screening for and addressing age-related disease. The prevalence of various age-related diseases varies by disease.

- Depending on the study criteria, 28% to 68% of dogs older than 9 years show clinical signs consistent with cognitive dysfunction.[10]
- Chronic kidney disease (CKD) occurs at a rate of 0.3% to 1.5% within the general dog population but at a rate of 10% to 15% in aged dogs.[11–13]
- Cancer may account for approximately 20% of dog deaths at 5 years and up to 40% to 50% of dogs aged 10 to 16 years.[14]
- According to survey data, dogs with arthritis, skin tumors, periodontal disease, and heart murmur are likely to be those older than 10 years.[4]
- Arthritis is particularly common, with many as 20% of adult dogs being affected in one study.[15]

The incidence of disease in this population likely represents a continuum from normal adult to normal aging changes to disease caused by aging changes; however, different organ systems likely progress along the continuum at different rates as not all

---

Box 1
Approach to nutritional assessment and therapy for aging dogs

- Detailed assessment of:
  - Patient
  - Diet
  - Feeding management
- Adjustments in either/both:
  - Diet
  - Feeding management
- Aging affects patients, but adjustments in diet/feeding management should be made accordingly and on an individualized basis.

Box 2
Factors to consider when assessing the aged dog

- Assessment of body condition: Is the dog overweight or underweight?
- Is the dog eating appropriate amounts of a balanced diet?
- Have all possible nutritionally-relevant aging changes been accommodated?
  - Intake/sensory
    - Assess whether the dog can appropriately prehend, masticate, and swallow food. The assessment of oral health and swallowing ability is indicated in underweight patients.
    - Assess whether the diet is palatable to the dog. Measures such as adding water to kibble and warming food may help increase food intake.
  - Mobility and access to food source
    - Assess whether standing to eat is possible, if the dog can ambulate to find food, and/or other pets are hindering access to food.
  - Mobility and exercise
    - Exercise may encourage an ideal body condition and may be helpful in the management of osteoarthritis.
    - Activity may also positively impact sarcopenia, and exploration of new environments provides mental stimulation. Even in minimally ambulatory dogs, sniffing is an important need; this pleasurable activity should be provided.

---

of the organs fail because of aging changes at the same time (**Fig. 1**). Both normal aging changes and age-related diseases are potentially responsive to nutritional intervention. Consideration of these issues separately is warranted, as dietary strategies to manage them (or at least commercial diets designed to manage them) may be contradictory and should not be applied universally (**Table 1**).

PHYSIOLOGIC CHANGES ASSOCIATED WITH AGING

Changes associated with aging may be physiologic or pathologic. There are many important physiologic changes that occur normally with aging, including changes in body composition and metabolic rates as well as declines in special senses.

Other concurrent changes may be pathologic and are associated with nutritional status; however, both expected and pathologic changes may be amenable to nutritional interventions. In addition, as this population is more likely to be afflicted with various diseases more common in aged dogs, attention to any process that is potentially nutritionally responsive is warranted.

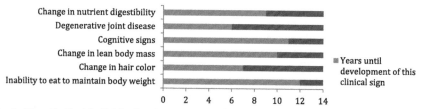

Fig. 1. Hypothetical individualized assessment of aging. A dog would be considered senior or geriatric after it had met a specified milestone or number of milestones. The veterinarian determines which milestones are assessed, the relative degree of signs, and the indications for specific intervention.

Table 1
Considerations for alterations of nutrient intake for healthy senior dogs

Key Nutrient	Alteration	Rationale
Energy	Increase or decrease	Senior dogs have overall decreased energy requirements, but older dogs are also more likely to be underweight.
Protein	Increase, unless evidence of disease indicating protein reduction	The protein requirements of senior dogs increase with age because of the increased protein turnover.
Fat	Increase or decrease	Senior dogs have no alteration in fat digestibility with age, so fat should increase or decrease as needed to affect the energy density of the diet.
Long-chain omega-3 polyunsaturated fatty acids	No alteration or increase	Evidence is not conclusive, but long-chain omega-3 polyunsaturated fatty acids may be beneficial in delaying the onset and progression of several physiologic aging changes as well as improving clinical signs and delaying progression of age-related disease.
Antioxidants	No alteration or increase	Evidence is not conclusive, but several studies indicate that dietary enrichment with a variety of antioxidant cocktails improves cognitive function. Clear dose-response relationships have not been elucidated.

Impact of Aging on Nutrient Absorption

Some of the changes associated with aging directly affect digestion and assimilation of food. These changes include anatomic changes, such as histologic gut morphology, whereby older dogs have been shown to have less duodenal villus surface area, lower jejunal villus height, and greater colonic crypt depth.[16] Multiple functional changes including some effects on nutrient digestibility have also been documented, although findings among different studies are not consistent, and most reports do not support significant changes with aging.[17–20] One study reported higher interindividual variability in older versus younger dogs,[17] so this may partly explain conflicting results. In addition, there may be an impact of dietary adaption or of absolute age of the dogs, in the case of using very young dogs. For example, one study reported increased digestibility of dry matter, organic matter, and fat in older (11–12 years old) beagles compared with approximately 5-month old puppies; this effect disappeared after 10 months on the diets, which may have reflected an increased digestive efficiency in the puppies once they reached 1 year of age.[21]

No studies have reported a decreased digestive efficiency in geriatric dogs. There are several reports of no effect of age on nutrient digestibility in dogs, including investigations of macronutrient[17–20] and mineral digestibility (calcium, phosphorus, magnesium, zinc, copper, iron, potassium, and sodium).[19] Other studies have shown modest increases in nutrient digestibility in adult dogs of various ages. One study showed small increases in ash, protein, and fat digestion in aged dogs; however, these researchers also reported that comparisons done under other conditions (different time periods and using different numbers of dogs on different diets) resulted in no differences.[19] In addition, results have been variable for fat digestibility, with some studies reporting increases for older dogs and others reporting no difference.[9] One study[18] reporting increased fat digestibility in older (8–15 years) dogs used very small numbers (4 dogs in each group) and compared these dogs with puppies of 7 months of age. Given that more recent studies have documented a similar effect followed by no difference between age groups and that digestive efficiency seems to increase during growth in dogs, this may reflect physiologic changes in the puppies rather than in the older dogs.

Other functional effects of canine aging, such as diminished hydrochloric acid production and bile acid secretion, have been noted; however, as with humans, these have little overall significance.[22] Additionally, changes in salivary glands, small intestine, liver, and pancreas have been documented in aged dogs. These changes likely reflect the general organ degeneration associated with aging[9] and, because dogs have adequate digestive functional reserve, may not be clinically relevant.[20]

In summary, there are potentially important physiologic effects of aging on the digestive process; however, most studies report no differences in nutrient absorption when comparing young adult with geriatric dogs.

Impact of Aging on Gut Microbiota

Aging may also affect intestinal bacterial populations and concentrations of their products; whether a change in luminal concentration of bacterial products is detectable would also be a function of its rates of absorption or degradation. Studies have produced variable results on this subject, with most detecting both change and no change between adult and senior dogs, depending on parameter assessed.

It has been reported that gastric and small intestinal bacterial populations are similar between old and young dogs but that the colon of old dogs have lower concentrations of *Bacteroides*, Eubacteria, *Peptostreptococci*, *Bifidobacteria*, lactobacilli, and staphylococci and higher concentrations of a clostridial variety compared with young dogs fed the same diet.[23] With respect to *Bacteroides*, these findings were confirmed by another diet-controlled study[24]; but no differences were found for lactobacilli and *Bifidobacteria*. Conversely, there is one report of a study that found the opposite with respect to lactobacilli, with a 118% increase in old dogs compared with young dogs fed the same diet.[25] In addition, these researchers reported that total anaerobic bacteria in colonic contents of senior dogs increased 41% and *Clostridium* spp increased 344% in old dogs compared with young adults.[25]

Although one study[26] found no difference in fecal bacterial populations (when assessed as total aerobes, total anaerobes, *Bifidobacterium*, *Lactobacillus*, *Clostridium*, and *Escherichia coli*) between old and young dogs, there were lower fecal concentrations of bacterial products (butyrate, histamine, agmatine, and spermine) and higher fecal pH in old dogs. This difference in bacterial product concentrations and pH implies an undetected change in bacterial populations, differences in bacterial metabolism between dogs of different ages, or differences in intestinal absorption or degradation of these compounds.

Of course, a major limitation of many studies investigating microbial populations in the gastrointestinal (GI) tract is the reliance on fecal samples as a surrogate for characterization of microbes in situ. Achieving accurate assessments of microbiota populations at various regions within the GI tract remains a challenge. Further, the use of different technological tools to assess populations of GI microbes (culture techniques, DNA quantification, and characterization) among published studies further complicates interpretation. As speciation of microflora becomes more precise and comparisons of microbial populations becomes more accessible, trends in alteration of gut microflora with aging will likely become more clearly defined and can enable meaningful conclusions.

Impact of Aging on the Brain

Although this occurs in many tissue types, given the unique composition, metabolism, and physiology of the brain, the oxidative nature of aging is perhaps easiest to demonstrate in the context of the brain. Brain aging in dogs is a complex set of phenomena with both similarities and differences when compared with the process in humans. Oxidative changes are particularly detrimental in the brain because of 3 factors: its high metabolic rate, which results in production of reactive oxygen species, particularly in older individuals[27]; its high lipid content, which increases its susceptibility to oxidative damage; and its limited regenerative capacity, which makes the damage more apparent.[28,29] Aging has also inconsistently been shown to affect antioxidant status, with increases, no change, or decreases in specific antioxidant compounds.[30,31] Thus, any intervention that alters any of these 3 processes may affect progression of cognitive dysfunction. Additionally, the brain's glucose metabolism becomes less efficient with age, which contributes to increased production of reactive oxygen species,[32] so providing alternative fuel sources may be beneficial.

Impact of Aging on Immune Health

Several parameters related to the immune system have also been shown to be altered by the aging process, both with respect to cellular and humoral immunity. Decreases in total white blood cells and immature neutrophils[33] and lymphocytes[26] and increased numbers of mature neutrophils[33] are reported. In vitro, mononuclear cells of older dogs were less responsive to stimuli than those of young dogs; however, there was no difference in production of inflammatory mediators in response to lipopolysaccharide between young and old dogs.[34] In addition, it is generally recognized that an increased risk of infectious disease is a feature of young dogs rather than senior ones. When in vivo assessment of responsiveness was assessed as a delayed-type hypersensitivity response, age did not affect responses.[34]

Old dogs are also reported to have increased concentrations of immunoglobulin G[33] and either decreased antibody production[34] or no difference[35] in antibody titer in response to foreign antigens.

Impact of Aging on Gene Expression

Alterations in gene expression in specific tissues occur with age. Within the liver, aging affected 1.7% of nearly 14,000 genes expressed by hepatic tissue, with more pronounced gene expression alterations in dogs fed a higher-fat and higher-protein animal-based diet compared with a lower-fat and lower-protein plant-based diet.[36] Within adipose tissue, aging effects were more minimal, with alteration of expression of genes related to immune function and inflammatory response.[37] The clinical effects of these findings, if any, remain unclear.

Impact of Aging on Special Senses and Metabolic Flexibility

Senior dogs may also have alterations in several areas of ability to detect changes in and response to their environment. Although not proven in dogs, geriatric humans have shown a decreased ability to respond to dehydration[38]; this same finding seems to be likely in dogs.[9] Decreased sensory capabilities, such as olfaction, hearing, and taste, may contribute to a decrease in the influence of the cephalic stage of feeding.[9] This decrease could cause alterations in digestive physiology, as feed-forward signaling within the GI tract would be lost or diminished.

Metabolic responses to feeding are also altered in geriatric dogs, with basal insulin concentrations, insulin peak, and insulin change from baseline all increasing with age[39,40] and decreasing insulin response with age in another study.[33] Older dogs took longer to absorb glucose from meals and longer for serum glucose concentrations to return to baseline.[40] Hormonal response to ghrelin, an appetite-stimulating hormone, was reduced in old compared with young adult dogs.[41] Decreased ghrelin response may contribute to decreased appetite in some older animals,[9] in addition to the impacts of decreased olfaction and taste.

NUTRITIONAL MANAGEMENT OF PHYSIOLOGIC AGING CHANGES

The ideal nutritional profile of a diet for senior dogs is not agreed on, and regulatory standards for any nutrients have not been established. Several pet food manufacturers offer senior canine diets; but given the lack of regulatory guidelines, there is wide variation in energy density and concentrations of specific nutrients as well as inclusion of other potentially functional nutrients, such as chondroprotective supplements.

Energy

In general, the energy requirements of older dogs decrease with age.[42–44] The magnitude of the decrease has been reported to be approximately 20%[20,44–46] but may range up to 50%.[47] One reason for the decline is associated with an age-related decline in lean body mass (LBM)[48] because the primary driver of resting energy requirement is LBM,[49] and LBM declines with age[50] with a concurrent increase in body fat mass.[51–53]

However, other causes may also be involved, as decreased lean body mass has not been noted in all cases of older dogs with decreased maintenance energy requirement.[47] Certainly age- or disease-related decline in activity will further reduce energy requirements. If energy intake is not adjusted to maintain ideal BCS and compensate for decreased energy needs, the risk of obesity will increase. It is important to monitor body condition in order to prevent obesity because this condition exacerbates many age-related diseases. For obese-prone older dogs, the use of diets with lower energy density and higher concentrations of fiber may be useful to promote satiety and an ideal body condition.[54,55] It has been shown that, in Labrador retrievers, caloric restriction to an intake that sustains an ideal body condition score over an individual's lifetime results in significantly increased longevity.[53]

Despite increasing rates of obesity and a recognized lower energy requirement, overall, a higher prevalence of geriatric dogs classified as underweight compared with other age groups has also been reported.[56] Further, in some populations, the body condition score may be negatively correlated with age.[57] In some cases, this may be related to an underlying undiagnosed or uncontrolled age-related disease. An individualized approach is indicated with regard to both assessment and nutritional management plans because it cannot be assumed that all dogs older than a certain age need caloric reduction or increase.

Protein

Protein requirements to maintain nitrogen balance actually increase with age[58]; this is related to an increase in protein turnover, which results in increased nitrogen excretion.[48,58]

This increased protein requirement does not seem to be an effect of decreased digestibility; in fact, as discussed earlier, several studies support a static or increased digestive efficiency for protein.[19,21] However, there is an age-related decline in protein synthesis[59] and increased protein turnover in older animals.[58] Unless medically indicated, older dogs do not benefit from dietary protein restriction[60,61]; in fact, healthy adult animals show a reduction in function with dietary protein restriction.[62,63] Because older pets have a higher requirement for dietary protein, a reduction in intake further widens the gap between need and provision and is likely to be even more detrimental than in younger animals.[48] In addition, if caloric intake is decreased to manage weight gain, the proportion of energy provided as protein should be increased.[48,64]

Phosphorus

Although phosphorus restriction has been shown to slow progression of disease in dogs with CKD,[65] there is no evidence that this is effective in the prevention of the development of CKD. Restriction is not warranted unless and until CKD is documented, which underscores the importance of regular screening and assessment of dogs for risk factors for CKD as well as other diseases.

It is important to note that although commercial diets marketed for senior dogs are often assumed to be lower in protein and phosphorus compared with other maintenance diets,[5] they are not formulated to address CKD. For example, in the United States, most senior diets are formulated to meet the Association of American Feed Control Officials (AAFCO) Dog Food Nutrient Profiles for adult dogs, which specifies a minimum of 1.4 g phosphorus/1000 kcal; however, one study assessing 37 diets marketed for senior dogs reported a wide range of phosphorus concentrations, up to almost 3 times the minimum (all diets contained phosphorus below the maximum per AAFCO).[5] Senior diets are not appropriately phosphorus restricted for dogs with CKD, although they are adequate for healthy adults and seniors.

Sodium

Healthy dogs with access to water are able to tolerate a wide range of sodium intakes.[66] There has been no correlation between blood pressure and sodium intakes in dogs with experimentally induced CKD.[67] Further, sodium restriction even in dogs with primary hypertension, which is rare, seems to have minimal effect[68]; other studies have shown that restriction activates the renin-angiotensin-aldosterone system and may contribute to hypertension in some individuals.[69] The current recommendations are to avoid excessive sodium intake in hypertensive dogs without specifically implementing restriction[70]; of course, the terms *excessive* and *restriction* are subjective unless defined. Typically, *restriction* would be defined as intake less than the National Research Council-recommended allowance of 200 mg sodium per 1000 kcal, and *excess* exceeds the safe upper limit of 3.75 g sodium per 1000 kcal.[66]

NUTRITIONAL MANAGEMENT OF SELECTED AGE-RELATED DISEASES

Several other nutrients and other compounds may be of interest because of their impact on cognitive dysfunction, oxidative damage and/or the immune system, and degenerative joint disease.

Nutritional Intervention for Cognitive Dysfunction

Antioxidants

The combination of environmental enrichment and dietary enrichment with antioxidants has been reported to improve clinical signs related to recognition, sleep patterns, social interaction, house soiling, and owner- and veterinarian-perceived behavior score in dogs with cognitive dysfunction.[71] In another study, dogs fed a diet enriched with a different antioxidant blend including vitamin C, vitamin E, carnitine, lipoic acid, glutathione, and a variety of fruit and vegetables showed improved learning, ability to perform specific tasks, agility, and recognition compared with dogs fed a control diet,[29] similar to findings in other species.[72–75]

Long-chain omega-3 polyunsaturated fatty acids

Besides antioxidants, other nutritional interventions may also contribute to improvement in clinical signs of cognitive dysfunction. The brain has a high concentration of long-chain omega-3 polyunsaturated fatty acids (PUFA), and supplementation with these PUFA has been shown to be beneficial in brain development in dogs.[76] Dietary supplementation with these PUFA could be beneficial with respect to brain aging; this has not been assessed in dogs, but results from other species show some benefit to cognitive function.[77,78]

Alternative fuel sources

In addition to glucose, neural tissues are able to use lactate[79,80] and ketones[32] as energy sources, which contributes to exercise's beneficial effect on brain function.[81] Medium-chain triglycerides are metabolized to ketones by the liver. Ketones are able to cross the blood-brain barrier and can result in up to 20% sparing of glucose[82] for the brain's energy metabolism.[83] This supplementation also increased the concentration of long-chain omega-3 PUFA in the brains of old dogs,[82] making the lipid composition of the brain more like that of a young dog. In another study, medium-chain triglyceride–supplemented dogs demonstrated improved mitochondrial function, redox status, and fewer amyloid protein deposits.[32] Further, supplementation with medium-chain triglycerides resulted in improved cognitive performance in old dogs, compared with unsupplemented controls.[83]

Nutritional Intervention for Declining Immunity

Many aging changes occur as a result of oxidative damage at a cellular and subcellular level.[84] In addition to the brain, the unique physiology of the immune system makes it particularly vulnerable to oxidative changes.[85] Like other aspects of aging,[86,87] oxidative damage plays a role in declining immunity with age; but this decline can be affected nutritionally. The exact mechanisms by which specific compounds exert their effects are not fully elucidated, making it also not possible to define specific dosages or ratios at which these nutrients should be provided at this time.

Dietary enrichment with a combination of antioxidants and mitochondrial cofactors (vitamin E, L-carnitine, lipoic acid, vitamin C, and a variety of fruits and vegetables) in conjunction with behavioral enrichment increased neutrophil phagocytosis in dogs across a range of ages.[88] As a follow-up to this study, it was shown that the dietary inclusion of vitamins C and E, but not the addition of dietary fish oil, caused this improvement in neutrophil-mediated bacterial killing.[89]

Although not an essential nutrient for dogs, vitamin C (ascorbic acid) may become relevant to changes occurring in senior dogs. In rats, vitamin C recycling decreases with age, so it is theorized that vitamin C may become conditionally essential in aged individuals.[90,91] Dogs and cats have a decreased synthetic capacity for vitamin C compared with most other mammals.[92] If the findings in rats are also true for dogs, increasing the vitamin C intake of senior dogs may be reasonable. One study that assessed the effect of vitamin C supplementation in dogs younger than 2.5 and older than 7 years found no effect of vitamin C supplementation on antioxidant status or immunologic parameters.[93]

Vitamin E improved cellular immunity, as measured by delayed-type hypersensitivity skin test, but had no effect on humoral immunity, as measured by antibody production in response to foreign antigens in older dogs.[94]

Vitamin A supplementation in old dogs resulted in an increased CD4+/CD8+ ratio, increased proliferation of peripheral blood mononuclear cells in response to stimulus, and an increase in delayed-type hypersensitivity response to one but not other antigens.[95] The effects of supplementation with a related compound, lutein, on the canine immune system has been studied in young but not older dogs; this study found that lutein supplementation enhanced some measures of cell-mediated and humoral immunity.[96]

Dietary supplementation with lipoic acid has been shown to promote a favorable ratio of reduced/oxidized glutathione in the white blood cells of adult dogs.[97]

It must be kept in mind that findings of measurable antioxidant response, in vitro or even in vivo, when assessed by trained observers may or may not translate to a relevant functional difference in pets.

Nutritional Intervention for Degenerative Joint Disease

Management of body fat and muscle mass

Owners of senior and geriatric dogs should be aware of their dog's current intake and receive advice on appropriate amounts to feed in order to either attain or maintain their dog's ideal body weight, particularly because the dog's caloric needs may be changing during this life stage. Because obesity/overweight not only exacerbates clinical signs of degenerative joint disease (DJD) but may also contribute to the development of DJD, its prevention is indicated.[64] In addition, it is now well understood that obesity is a proinflammatory condition[98] with increased oxidative stress.[99] Weight loss has been shown to improve veterinarian-assessed lameness in arthritic dogs.[100] Given its association with obesity and increased prevalence in older populations, hypothyroidism should be ruled out in overweight senior dogs.

Maintenance of appropriate LBM and prevention of sarcopenia is warranted in senior dogs. Promoting daily exercise and the use of a balanced diet that meets the requirements for protein and other nutrients will help avoid adipose gain while preventing loss of muscle mass; the goal is to delay the onset or progression of disease.[64]

Long-chain omega-3 PUFA

Of the nonpharmacologic/nutraceutical treatments for DJD, the most evidence for efficacy exists for use of long-chain omega-3 PUFA found in marine oils. Supplementation with fish oils has shown clinical improvement and decreases in synovial inflammation and osteophyte formation,[101] improved weight bearing,[64,102–106] and owner-reported reduced clinical signs[106,107] in arthritic dogs. The recommended doses vary; one researcher recommended 2.5 g of long-chain omega-3 PUFA from fish oil per 1000 kcal.[64] Although there seems to be a therapeutic benefit from this treatment, there is also evidence for potential harm, with old dogs fed long-chain omega-3 PUFA showing increased measures of lipid peroxidation and suppressed cell-mediated immunity, though these findings may be partially explained by inadequate concurrent vitamin E intake in this study.[108]

Green-lipped mussel extract

Green-lipped mussel extract has also been promoted as beneficial in DJD. Efficacy of supplementation with green-lipped mussel extract seems to depend on the method of assessment, with improvements in overall arthritis scores and joint pain and swelling but no difference in joint crepitus and range of motion between supplemented and unsupplemented dogs with arthritis.[109,110] Green-lipped mussel extract supplementation was reported to provide improvement in subjective and objective assessments of DJD clinical signs as determined by pet owners and veterinarians that were intermediate between no treatment and carprofen treatment.[111] However, in another study,[112] neither owner- nor veterinarian-assessed improvement was seen in adult arthritic dogs compared with the control.

Glucosamine and chondroitin

Similar to data in humans,[113,114] veterinary data are conflicting on the efficacy of glucosamine and chondroitin supplementation[115]; some of this may be caused by variation in dosage, form, and delivery. These 2 compounds are frequently administered and assessed for efficacy together because they are expected to be synergistic[116]; there are no published studies evaluating glucosamine supplementation alone in dogs. Although one study has shown clinical benefit to supplementation with this combination as measured by veterinarian assessment,[117] others[112,118] showed no effect compared with placebo.

Other nutraceuticals

Various other compounds have been evaluated for effect in dogs with DJD. Arthritic dogs treated with turmeric extract showed no improvement in weight bearing as assessed by force plate or owner evaluation but showed improvement in veterinarian evaluation.[119] An uncontrolled study of Boswellia resin extract supplementation[120] in arthritic dogs showed subjective improvement in lameness. Special milk protein concentrate supplementation in arthritic dogs resulted in owner-perceived but not veterinarian-assessed improvement.[121] Elk velvet antler was shown to improve subjective and objective assessments of clinical signs of DJD in adult dogs.[122] Avocado and soy unsaponifiables have in vitro effects suggesting they may be helpful in managing DJD.[123,124] A placebo-controlled canine in vivo trial using avocado and soy unsaponifiables in dogs with experimentally induced DJD showed decreased severity of histologic lesions in treated dogs[123]; though heterogeneous, results from human trials suggest a possible clinical benefit.[125]

REASSESSMENT AND TREATMENT ADJUSTMENT

Regardless of the specific condition being managed or prevented, treatment plan goals and monitoring guidelines should be established with consideration for the expected clinical effects, as these may be subtle or not immediately apparent. A review of the current literature related to the particular intervention is warranted to establish this. It is also important to establish appropriate expectations with pet owners, which will allow for reassessment and adjustment as needed and provide improved care to the patients. Several of the aforementioned possible nutraceutical treatments, particularly for DJD, have not been thoroughly researched; as with any treatment, a positive effect is not guaranteed. Dietary supplements are not of uniform quality and consistency, and the risks associated with continued use of a substance that is not showing clinical effects in an individual patient may outweigh the potential benefits.

DISCUSSION

Although the formulation of an algorithm to diagnose, assess, and accommodate and/or treat both physiologic aging changes and age-related disease would be ideal, there is sufficient interindividual variation in aging to make this goal not only impossible but also not highly useful. For a given patient, the parameters related to aging that are of most concern are a function of the patient's signalment and lifestyle as well as current health status. For example, the onset of DJD of the elbow is unfortunate for any dog. However, this has a greater negative impact for a large-breed or working dog, as opposed to a smaller or strictly companion animal, particularly if its owner also has a relatively sedentary lifestyle. For this reason, an individualized set of criteria would ideally be prescribed to assess a patient as it ages. Such an approach would require the following:

1. During a routine examination of a mature adult dog, the veterinarian and pet owner would define criteria/milestones relevant to the patient's well-being and its ability to function in its normal capacity. Which milestones mark transitions from adult to senior to geriatric would also be determined at this time.
2. The age at which the patient achieves the relevant milestones is recorded as the patient ages. The patient would be considered to advance from adult to senior to geriatric as it achieves specific milestones or a certain number of milestones.
3. The veterinarian would use this system to recommend certain individualized assessments based on the patient's progression through the aging process. Because the terms *aging* and *old/getting older* may mean different things to different pet owners, this provides an objective picture of a patient's *physiologic age*. A hypothetical example of this is demonstrated in **Fig. 1**. Of course, classification of an individual as *adult* versus *senior* versus *geriatric* has limited clinical implication in terms of comparing one patient to another, as not all animals in the same category will display the same clinical manifestations of their age and, thus, will require different interventions. This classification strategy is, however, a tool to illustrate to the patient's owners its clinical status and serve as a justification for diagnostic and treatment recommendations. Further, it may serve as a reminder of a patient's disability status at a given point in time, such that if therapy yields an improvement, the efficacy of therapy in that patient would be highlighted.

It should be kept in mind that each of the nutraceuticals discussed earlier for the management of age-related diseases have either an incompletely assessed efficacy or have conflicting results between subjective and objective assessments or between studies. The decision to use or not to use these in an individual patient should take into consideration the potential risks and benefits in addition to the consideration of how well study data generalizes to the individual being treated.

SUMMARY

As dogs age, they experience a wide variety of metabolic changes that affect both structure and function. These changes may consist of normal, physiologic aging changes or may manifest as age-related disease. Screening for these changes via routine physical examination and laboratory assessment is critical to affecting the processes at stages where their courses may be altered. Accommodating the specific changes observed in each individual, rather than adopting a generic senior dog approach, will allow tailoring a patient's treatment plan to the individual's needs. Demonstrating this to pet owners will also likely increase compliance and further improve care for patients.

REFERENCES

1. American Veterinary Medical Association. Total pet ownership and pet population. US pet ownership & demographics sourcebook. Schamburg (IL): AVMA Membership & Field Services; 2012. p. 1–49.
2. Laflamme DP, Abood SK, Fascetti AJ, et al. Pet feeding practices of dog and cat owners in the United States and Australia. J Am Vet Med Assoc 2008;232: 687–94.

3. Banfield Pet Hospital State of Pet Health 2013 Report. 2013. Available at: http://www.stateofpethealth.com/Content/pdf/Banfield-State-of-Pet-Health-Report_2013.pdf. Accessed October 21, 2013.

4. Banfield Pet Hospital State of Pet Health 2012 Report. 2012. Available at: http://www.stateofpethealth.com/Content/pdf/Banfield-State-of-Pet-Health-Report_2012.pdf. Accessed October 30, 2013.

5. Hutchinson D, Freeman LM, Schreiner KE, et al. Survey of opinions about nutritional requirements of senior dogs and analysis of nutrient profiles of commercially available diets for senior dogs. Int J Appl Res Vet Med 2011; 9:68–79.

6. Adams VJ, Evans KM, Sampson J, et al. Methods and mortality results of a health survey of purebred dogs in the UK. J Small Anim Pract 2010;51:512–24.

7. Fick LJ, Fick GH, Li Z, et al. Telomere length correlates with life span of dog breeds. Cell Rep 2012;2:1530–6.

8. Epstein M, Kuehn NF, Landsberg G, et al. AAHA senior care guidelines for dogs and cats. J Am Anim Hosp Assoc 2005;41:81–91.

9. Fahey GC Jr, Barry KA, Swanson KS. Age-related changes in nutrient utilization by companion animals. Annu Rev Nutr 2008;28:425–45.

10. Landsberg GM, Nichol J, Araujo JA. Cognitive dysfunction syndrome: a disease of canine and feline brain aging. Vet Clin North Am Small Anim Pract 2012;42: 749–68, vii.

11. Bartges JW. Chronic kidney disease in dogs and cats. Vet Clin North Am Small Anim Pract 2012;42:669–92, vi.

12. O'Neill DG, Elliott J, Church DB, et al. Chronic kidney disease in dogs in UK veterinary practices: prevalence, risk factors, and survival. J Vet Intern Med 2013; 27:814–21.

13. Polzin DJ, Osborne CA, Adams LD, et al. Dietary management of canine and feline chronic renal failure. Vet Clin North Am Small Anim Pract 1989;19:539–60.

14. Bronson RT. Variation in age at death of dogs of different sexes and breeds. Am J Vet Res 1982;43:2057–9.

15. Aragon CL, Hofmeister EH, Budsberg SC. Systematic review of clinical trials of treatments for osteoarthritis in dogs. J Am Vet Med Assoc 2007;230:514–21.

16. Kuzmuk KN, Swanson KS, Tappenden KA, et al. Diet and age affect intestinal morphology and large bowel fermentative end-product concentrations in senior and young adult dogs. J Nutr 2005;135:1940–5.

17. Buffington CA. Lack of effect of age on digestibility of protein, fat, and dry matter in beagle dogs. In: Burger I, Rivers J, editors. Nutrition of the dog and cat. 1st edition. New York: Cambridge University Press; 1989. p. 397.

18. Lloyd LE, McCay CM. The use of chromic oxide in digestibility and balance studies with dogs. J Nutr 1954;53:613–22.

19. Sheffy BE, Williams AJ, Zimmer JF, et al. Nutrition and metabolism of the geriatric dog. Cornell Vet 1985;75:324–47.

20. Taylor EJ, Adams C, Neville R. Some nutritional aspects of ageing in dogs and cats. Proc Nutr Soc 1995;54:645–56.

21. Swanson KS, Kuzmuk KN, Schook LB, et al. Diet affects nutrient digestibility, hematology, and serum chemistry of senior and weanling dogs. J Anim Sci 2004; 82:1713–24.

22. Mosier JE. Effect of aging on body systems of the dog. Vet Clin North Am Small Anim Pract 1989;19:1–12.

23. Benno Y, Nakao H, Uchida K, et al. Impact of the advances in age on the gastrointestinal microflora of beagle dogs. J Vet Med Sci 1992;54:703–6.

24. Simpson JM, Martineau B, Jones WE, et al. Characterization of fecal bacterial populations in canines: effects of age, breed and dietary fiber. Microb Ecol 2002;44:186–97.

25. Kearns RJ, Hayek MG, Sunvold GD. Microbial changes in aged dogs. In: Reinhart GA, Carey DP, editors. 1998 Iams Nutrition Symposium proceedings: recent advances in canine and feline nutrition. Wilmington OH: Orange Frazer Press; 1998. p. 337–51.

26. Gomes MO, Beraldo MC, Putarov TC, et al. Old beagle dogs have lower faecal concentrations of some fermentation products and lower peripheral lymphocyte counts than young adult beagles. Br J Nutr 2011;106(Suppl 1): S187–90.

27. Beckman KB, Ames BN. The free radical theory of aging matures. Physiol Rev 1998;78:547–81.

28. Manteca X. Nutrition and behavior in senior dogs. Top Companion Anim Med 2011;26:33–6.

29. Roudebush P, Zicker SC, Cotman CW, et al. Nutritional management of brain aging in dogs. J Am Vet Med Assoc 2005;227:722–8.

30. Stowe HD, Lawler DF, Kealy RD. Antioxidant status of pair-fed Labrador retrievers is affected by diet restriction and aging. J Nutr 2006;136:1844–8.

31. Moyer KL, Trepanier LA. Erythrocyte glutathione and plasma cysteine concentrations in young versus old dogs. J Am Vet Med Assoc 2009;234:95–9.

32. Studzinski CM, MacKay WA, Beckett TL, et al. Induction of ketosis may improve mitochondrial function and decrease steady-state amyloid-beta precursor protein (APP) levels in the aged dog. Brain Res 2008;1226:209–17.

33. Strasser A, Niedermuller H, Hofecker G, et al. The effect of aging on laboratory values in dogs. Zentralbl Veterinarmed A 1993;40:720–30.

34. Kearns RJ, Hayek MG, Turek JJ, et al. Effect of age, breed and dietary omega-6 (n-6): omega-3 (n-3) fatty acid ratio on immune function, eicosanoid production, and lipid peroxidation in young and aged dogs. Vet Immunol Immunopathol 1999;69:165–83.

35. Greeley EH, Kealy RD, Ballam JM, et al. The influence of age on the canine immune system. Vet Immunol Immunopathol 1996;55:1–10.

36. Kil DY, Vester Boler BM, Apanavicius CJ, et al. Age and diet affect gene expression profiles in canine liver tissue. PLoS One 2010;5:e13319.

37. Swanson KS, Belsito KR, Vester BM, et al. Adipose tissue gene expression profiles of healthy young adult and geriatric dogs. Arch Anim Nutr 2009;63: 160–71.

38. Kenney WL, Chiu P. Influence of age on thirst and fluid intake. Med Sci Sports Exerc 2001;33:1524–32.

39. Larson BT, Lawler DF, Spitznagel EL Jr, et al. Improved glucose tolerance with lifetime diet restriction favorably affects disease and survival in dogs. J Nutr 2003;133:2887–92.

40. Hayek MG, Sunvold GD. Influence of age on glucose metabolism in the senior companion animal: implications for long-term senior health. In: Reinhart GA, Carey DP, editors. Recent advances in canine and feline nutrition. Wilmington, OH: Orange Frazer Press; 2000. p. 403–13.

41. Bhatti SF, Duchateau L, Van Ham LM, et al. Effects of growth hormone secretagogues on the release of adenohypophyseal hormones in young and old healthy dogs. Vet J 2006;172:515–25.

42. Harper EJ. Changing perspectives on aging and energy requirements: aging and energy intakes in humans, dogs and cats. J Nutr 1998;128:2623S–6S.

43. LaFlamme DP, Martineau B, Jones W, et al. Effect of age on maintenance energy requirements and apparent digestibility of canine diets. Comp Cont Educ Pract Vet 2000;22:113.

44. Kienzle E, Rainbird A. Maintenance energy requirement of dogs: what is the correct value for the calculation of metabolic body weight in dogs? J Nutr 1991;121: S39–40.

45. Finke MD. Evaluation of the energy requirements of adult kennel dogs. J Nutr 1991;121:S22–8.

46. Burger I. Updated feeding recommendations for the canine diet. Focus 1995; 5:32.

47. Speakman JR, van Acker A, Harper EJ. Age-related changes in the metabolism and body composition of three dog breeds and their relationship to life expectancy. Aging Cell 2003;2:265–75.

48. Laflamme DP. Nutrition for aging cats and dogs and the importance of body condition. Vet Clin North Am Small Anim Pract 2005;35:713–42.

49. Elia M. The inter-organ flux of substrates in fed and fasted man, as indicated by arterio-venous balance studies. Nutr Res Rev 1991;4:3–31.

50. Kealy RD. Factors influencing lean body mass in aging dogs. Comp Cont Educ Pract Vet 1998;21:34–7.

51. Meyer J, Stadtfeld G. Investigation on the body and organ structure of dogs. In: Anderson RS, editor. Nutrition of the dog and cat. Oxford (United Kingdom): Pergamon Press; 1980. p. 15–30.

52. Harper EJ. Changing perspectives on aging and energy requirements: aging, body weight and body composition in humans, dogs and cats. J Nutr 1998; 128:2627S–31S.

53. Kealy RD, Lawler DF, Ballam JM, et al. Effects of diet restriction on life span and age-related changes in dogs. J Am Vet Med Assoc 2002;220:1315–20.

54. Jewell DE, Toll PW. Effects of fiber on food intake in dogs. Vet Clin Nutr 1996;3: 115–8.

55. Laflamme DP. Understanding and managing obesity in dogs and cats. Vet Clin North Am Small Anim Pract 2006;36:1283–95, vii.

56. Armstrong PJ, Lund EM. Changes in body composition and energy balance with aging. Vet Clin Nutr 1996;3:83–7.

57. Donoghue S, Khoo L, Glickman LT, et al. Body condition and diet of relatively healthy older dogs. J Nutr 1991;121:S58–9.

58. Wannemacher RW Jr, McCoy JR. Determination of optimal dietary protein requirements of young and old dogs. J Nutr 1966;88:66–74.

59. Richardson A, Birchenall-Sparks MC. Age-related changes in protein synthesis. Rev Biol Res Aging 1983;1:255–73.

60. Finco DR, Brown SA, Crowell WA, et al. Effects of aging and dietary protein intake on uninephrectomized geriatric dogs. Am J Vet Res 1994;55: 1282–90.

61. Bovee KC. Mythology of protein restriction for dogs with reduced renal function. Comp Cont Educ Pract Vet 1999;21:15–20.

62. McMurray DN. Effect of moderate protein deficiency on immune function. Compend Contin Educ Vet 1999;21:21–4.

63. Yoshino K, Sakai K, Okada H, et al. IgE responses in mice fed moderate protein deficient and high protein diets. J Nutr Sci Vitaminol (Tokyo) 2003; 49:172–8.

64. Laflamme DP. Nutritional care for aging cats and dogs. Vet Clin North Am Small Anim Pract 2012;42:769–91, vii.

65. Brown SA, Crowell WA, Barsanti JA, et al. Beneficial effects of dietary mineral restriction in dogs with marked reduction of functional renal mass. J Am Soc Nephrol 1991;1:1169–79.

66. Minerals. In: National Research Council, editor. Nutrient requirements of dogs and cats. Washington, DC: National Academies Press; 2006. p. 159–61.

67. Greco DS, Lees GE, Dzendzel G, et al. Effects of dietary sodium intake on blood pressure measurements in partially nephrectomized dogs. Am J Vet Res 1994; 55:160–5.

68. Littman MP, Robertson JL, Bovee KC. Spontaneous systemic hypertension in dogs: five cases (1981-1983). J Am Vet Med Assoc 1988;193:486–94.

69. Pedersen HD, Koch J, Jensen AL, et al. Some effects of a low sodium diet high in potassium on the renin-angiotensin system and plasma electrolyte concentrations in normal dogs. Acta Vet Scand 1994;35:133–40.

70. Chandler ML. Pet food safety: sodium in pet foods. Top Companion Anim Med 2008;23:148–53.

71. Pop V, Head E, Hill MA, et al. Synergistic effects of long-term antioxidant diet and behavioral enrichment on beta-amyloid load and non-amyloidogenic processing in aged canines. J Neurosci 2010;30:9831–9.

72. Tchantchou F, Chan A, Kifle L, et al. Apple juice concentrate prevents oxidative damage and impaired maze performance in aged mice. J Alzheimers Dis 2005; 8:283–7.

73. Shenk JC, Liu J, Fischbach K, et al. The effect of acetyl-L-carnitine and R-alpha-lipoic acid treatment in ApoE4 mouse as a model of human Alzheimer's disease. J Neurol Sci 2009;283:199–206.

74. Sinha M, Saha A, Basu S, et al. Aging and antioxidants modulate rat brain levels of homocysteine and dehydroepiandrosterone sulphate (DHEA-S): implications in the pathogenesis of Alzheimer's disease. Neurosci Lett 2010;483:123–6.

75. Murakami K, Murata N, Ozawa Y, et al. Vitamin C restores behavioral deficits and amyloid-beta oligomerization without affecting plaque formation in a mouse model of Alzheimer's disease. J Alzheimers Dis 2011;26:7–18.

76. Heinemann KM, Bauer JE. Docosahexaenoic acid and neurologic development in animals. J Am Vet Med Assoc 2006;228:700–5, 655.

77. Boudrault C, Bazinet RP, Ma DW. Experimental models and mechanisms underlying the protective effects of n-3 polyunsaturated fatty acids in Alzheimer's disease. J Nutr Biochem 2009;20:1–10.

78. Denis I, Potier B, Vancassel S, et al. Omega-3 fatty acids and brain resistance to ageing and stress: body of evidence and possible mechanisms. Ageing Res Rev 2013;12:579–94.

79. Sanchez-Abarca LI, Tabernero A, Medina JM. Oligodendrocytes use lactate as a source of energy and as a precursor of lipids. Glia 2001;36:321–9.

80. Overgaard M, Rasmussen P, Bohm AM, et al. Hypoxia and exercise provoke both lactate release and lactate oxidation by the human brain. FASEB J 2012;26:3012–20.

81. Ide K, Horn A, Secher NH. Cerebral metabolic response to submaximal exercise. J Appl Physiol (1985) 1999;87:1604–8.

82. Taha AY, Henderson ST, Burnham WM. Dietary enrichment with medium chain triglycerides (AC-1203) elevates polyunsaturated fatty acids in the parietal cortex of aged dogs: implications for treating age-related cognitive decline. Neurochem Res 2009;34:1619–25.

83. Pan Y, Larson B, Araujo JA, et al. Dietary supplementation with medium-chain TAG has long-lasting cognition-enhancing effects in aged dogs. Br J Nutr 2010;103: 1746–54.

84. Harman D. Aging: a theory based on free radical and radiation chemistry. J Gerontol 1956;11:298–300.

85. Satyaraj E. Emerging paradigms in immunonutrition. Top Companion Anim Med 2011;26:25–32.

86. Head E. Oxidative damage and cognitive dysfunction: antioxidant treatments to promote healthy brain aging. Neurochem Res 2009;34:670–8.

87. Brown SA. Oxidative stress and chronic kidney disease. Vet Clin North Am Small Anim Pract 2008;38:157–66, vi.

88. Hall JA, Picton RA, Finneran PS, et al. Dietary antioxidants and behavioral enrichment enhance neutrophil phagocytosis in geriatric beagles. Vet Immunol Immunopathol 2006;113:224–33.

89. Hall JA, Chinn RM, Vorachek WR, et al. Influence of dietary antioxidants and fatty acids on neutrophil mediated bacterial killing and gene expression in healthy beagles. Vet Immunol Immunopathol 2011;139:217–28.

90. Lykkesfeldt J, Hagen TM, Vinarsky V, et al. Age-associated decline in ascorbic acid concentration, recycling, and biosynthesis in rat hepatocytes–reversal with (R)-alpha-lipoic acid supplementation. FASEB J 1998;12:1183–9.

91. Michels AJ, Joisher N, Hagen TM. Age-related decline of sodium-dependent ascorbic acid transport in isolated rat hepatocytes. Arch Biochem Biophys 2003; 410:112–20.

92. Chatterjee IB, Majumder AK, Nandi BK, et al. Synthesis and some major functions of vitamin C in animals. Ann N Y Acad Sci 1975;258:24–47.

93. Hesta M, Ottermans C, Krammer-Lukas S, et al. The effect of vitamin C supplementation in healthy dogs on antioxidative capacity and immune parameters. J Anim Physiol Anim Nutr (Berl) 2009;93:26–34.

94. Hall JA, Tooley KA, Gradin JL, et al. Effects of dietary n-6 and n-3 fatty acids and vitamin E on the immune response of healthy geriatric dogs. Am J Vet Res 2003; 64:762–72.

95. Kearns RJ, Loos KM, Chew BP, et al. The effect of age and dietary beta-carotene on immunological parameters in the dog. In: Reinhart RA, Carey DP, editors. Recent advances in canine and feline nutrition-volume III: 2000 Iams Nutrition Symposium Proceedings. Wilmington OH: Orange Frazer Press; 2000.

96. Kim HW, Chew BP, Wong TS, et al. Dietary lutein stimulates immune response in the canine. Vet Immunol Immunopathol 2000;74:315–27.

97. Zicker SC, Hagen TM, Joisher N, et al. Safety of long-term feeding of dl-alpha-lipoic acid and its effect on reduced glutathione:oxidized glutathione ratios in beagles. Vet Ther 2002;3:167–76.

98. German AJ. Barking up the wrong tree: what's the deal with obesity, adiponectin and inflammation in dogs? Vet J 2012;194:272–3.

99. De Marchi E, Baldassari F, Bononi A, et al. Oxidative stress in cardiovascular diseases and obesity: role of p66Shc and protein kinase C. Oxid Med Cell Longev 2013;2013:564961.

100. Impellizeri JA, Tetrick MA, Muir P. Effect of weight reduction on clinical signs of lameness in dogs with hip osteoarthritis. J Am Vet Med Assoc 2000;216:1089–91.

101. Bartges JW, Budsberg SC, Pazak HE. Effects of different n6:n3 fatty acid ratio diets on canine stifle osteoarthritis. Orthopedic Research Society 47th Annual Meeting. February 25-28, San Francisco, CA, 2001.

102. Roush JK, Cross AR, Renberg WC. Effects of feeding a high omega-3 fatty acid diet on serum fatty acid profiles and force plate analysis in dogs with osteoarthritis. Vet Surg 2005;34.

103. Hansen RA, Harris MA, Pluhar GE, et al. Fish oil decreases matrix metalloproteinases in knee synovia of dogs with inflammatory joint disease. J Nutr Biochem 2008;19:101–8.
104. Fritsch DA, Allen TA, Dodd CE, et al. A multicenter study of the effect of dietary supplementation with fish oil omega-3 fatty acids on carprofen dosage in dogs with osteoarthritis. J Am Vet Med Assoc 2010;236:535–9.
105. Roush JK, Cross AR, Renberg WC, et al. Evaluation of the effects of dietary supplementation with fish oil omega-3 fatty acids on weight bearing in dogs with osteoarthritis. J Am Vet Med Assoc 2010;236:67–73.
106. Moreau M, Troncy E, Del Castillo JR, et al. Effects of feeding a high omega-3 fatty acids diet in dogs with naturally occurring osteoarthritis. J Anim Physiol Anim Nutr (Berl) 2012;97:830–7.
107. Miller WH, Scott DW, Wellington TR. Treatment of dogs with hip arthritis with a fatty acid supplement. Canine Practice 1992;17:6–8.
108. Wander RC, Hall JA, Gradin JL, et al. The ratio of dietary (n-6) to (n-3) fatty acids influences immune system function, eicosanoid metabolism, lipid peroxidation and vitamin E status in aged dogs. J Nutr 1997;127:1198–205.
109. Bui LM, Bierer RL. Influence of green lipped mussels (Perna canaliculus) in alleviating signs of arthritis in dogs. Vet Ther 2001;2:101–11.
110. Bierer TL, Bui LM. Improvement of arthritic signs in dogs fed green-lipped mussel (Perna canaliculus). J Nutr 2002;132:1634S–6S.
111. Hielm-Bjorkman A, Tulamo RM, Salonen H, et al. Evaluating complementary therapies for canine osteoarthritis part i: green-lipped mussel (Perna canaliculus). Evid Based Complement Alternat Med 2009;6:365–73.
112. Dobenecker B, Beetz Y, Kienzle E. A placebo-controlled double-blind study on the effect of nutraceuticals (chondroitin sulfate and mussel extract) in dogs with joint diseases as perceived by their owners. J Nutr 2002;132:1690S–1S.
113. Ragle RL, Sawitzke AD. Nutraceuticals in the management of osteoarthritis: a critical review. Drugs Aging 2012;29:717–31.
114. Miller KL, Clegg DO. Glucosamine and chondroitin sulfate. Rheum Dis Clin North Am 2011;37:103–18.
115. Budsberg SC, Bartges JW. Nutrition and osteoarthritis in dogs: does it help? Vet Clin North Am Small Anim Pract 2006;36:1307–23, vii.
116. Jerosch J. Effects of glucosamine and chondroitin sulfate on cartilage metabolism in OA: outlook on other nutrient partners especially omega-3 fatty acids. Int J Rheumatol 2011;2011:969012.
117. McCarthy G, O'Donovan J, Jones B, et al. Randomised double-blind, positive-controlled trial to assess the efficacy of glucosamine/chondroitin sulfate for the treatment of dogs with osteoarthritis. Vet J 2007;174:54–61.
118. Moreau M, Dupuis J, Bonneau NH, et al. Clinical evaluation of a nutraceutical, carprofen and meloxicam for the treatment of dogs with osteoarthritis. Vet Rec 2003;152:323–9.
119. Innes JF, Fuller CJ, Grover ER, et al. Randomised, double-blind, placebo-controlled parallel group study of P54FP for the treatment of dogs with osteoarthritis. Vet Rec 2003;152:457–60.
120. Reichling J, Schmokel H, Fitzi J, et al. Dietary support with Boswellia resin in canine inflammatory joint and spinal disease. Schweiz Arch Tierheilkd 2004;146:71–9.
121. Gingerich DA, Strobel JD. Use of client-specific outcome measures to assess treatment effects in geriatric, arthritic dogs: controlled clinical evaluation of a nutraceutical. Vet Ther 2003;4:376–86.

122. Moreau M, Dupuis J, Bonneau NH, et al. Clinical evaluation of a powder of quality elk velvet antler for the treatment of osteoarthrosis in dogs. Can Vet J 2004; 45:133–9.
123. Boileau C, Martel-Pelletier J, Caron J, et al. Protective effects of total fraction of avocado/soybean unsaponifiables on the structural changes in experimental dog osteoarthritis: inhibition of nitric oxide synthase and matrix metalloproteinase-13. Arthritis Res Ther 2009;11:R41.
124. Altinel L, Saritas ZK, Kose KC, et al. Treatment with unsaponifiable extracts of avocado and soybean increases TGF-beta1 and TGF-beta2 levels in canine joint fluid. Tohoku J Exp Med 2007;211:181–6.
125. Christensen R, Bartels EM, Astrup A, et al. Symptomatic efficacy of avocado-soybean unsaponifiables (ASU) in osteoarthritis (OA) patients: a meta-analysis of randomized controlled trials. Osteoarthritis Cartilage 2008;16:399–408.

Nutrition of Aging Cats

Dottie Laflamme, DVM, PhD[a],*,
Danièlle Gunn-Moore, BVM&S, PhD, MRCVS[b]

KEYWORDS

- Nutrition • Geriatric • Aging • Protein • Energy • Carbohydrates

KEY POINTS

- Changes in body weight, body condition score (BCS), and muscle mass can be especially meaningful in older cats: weight loss is often the first sign of disease in aging cats whereas loss of lean body mass (LBM) is a risk factor for increased mortality.
- Approximately 35% of geriatric cats have reduced ability to digest fat, and 20% have reduced ability to digest protein, which can contribute to weight loss and loss of lean body mass.
- To help compensate for undesired loss of weight or condition, many older cats may benefit from a highly palatable, highly digestible, energy-dense food that is offered in small amounts frequently: diets formulated for kittens can be a good option.
- Appropriate feeding management helps address some aspects of environmental enrichment and stress management, which can be particularly important in aging cats.
- Nutritional intervention can be beneficial for cats with many age-related diseases, but appropriate attention must be paid to total nutrient intake, calorie intake, and maintenance of body weight.

INTRODUCTION

Improvements in nutrition, health care, and management have led to many cats living to increasingly greater ages. Although the specific proportions differ among different studies, at least one-third of cats seen by veterinarians are 7 years of age or older, approximately 20% 10 years of age or older, and nearly 13% of cats are 12 years of age or older.[1,2]

Aging brings with it physiologic changes, even in apparently healthy cats. Some examples include a general decline in body and coat condition, failing senses (sight and smell), and altered behaviors.[3] Some changes are less obvious and may include decreased physiologic reserves and reduced functionality of the digestive, immune, renal, and other systems. Many of these physiologic changes, including changes in body weight and composition and in energy requirements, occur at predictable

[a] Nestlé Purina Research, Checkerboard Square, St. Louis, MO 63164, USA; [b] Royal (Dick) School of Veterinary Studies and The Roslin Institute, The University of Edinburgh, Easter Bush Campus, Roslin, EH25 9RG, Scotland
* Corresponding author.
E-mail address: Dorothy.laflamme@rd.nestle.com

Vet Clin Small Anim 44 (2014) 761–774
http://dx.doi.org/10.1016/j.cvsm.2014.03.001
0195-5616/14/$ – see front matter © 2014 Elsevier Inc. All rights reserved.

ages. Based on the onset of these changes, the feline population is divided into 4 distinctive life stages: growth; adult, for cats up to 6 years of age; mature, 7 until 12 years, a period when many cats become overweight or obese and are more likely to show evidence of chronic diseases; and geriatric, 12 years and above, when body weight tends to decrease progressively to below ideal and terminal conditions are increasingly recognized.[1,4,5] The focus of this article is the mature and geriatric age groups.

Chronologic age does not always match physiologic age. Thus, older cats must be cared for and fed based on their individual needs.

Management of aging cats can require changes in their care. Older cats often cope poorly with changes in their daily routine. Their response to stress is often to stop eating, hide, and/or alter their toileting habits. Illnesses or any change within the environment, the family, or even the diet can act as a source of stress. Because dietary changes can be stressful, it is important to make changes slowly. Sick cats should be stable, if possible, before introducing a new food to reduce stress and avoid food aversion. Environmental enrichment, which is important for all cats, should be specifically tailored for elderly cats (**Table 1**).

PHYSICAL AND NUTRITIONAL EVALUATION OF AGING CATS

Evaluation of aging cats begins with a good medical history, with open-ended questions about activity, attitudes, and behaviors, including changes in feeding, sleeping, litter box, and social behaviors.[3] Further questioning regarding bathroom habits can suggest problems with urinary or gastrointestinal function. A fecal score chart indicating stool softness and color can help identify diarrhea or constipation.

The physical examination should begin by observing a cat from a distance, assessing breathing patterns, gait, posture, and coordination, among other things. Evidence of physical weakness may be linked to nutritional deficiencies, such as potassium or thiamine. Evaluation of skin and hair coat can indicate underlying medical or nutritional

Table 1 Environmental adjustments for aging cats	
Key resource	All resources should be easily accessed. If an elderly cat has to walk too far for its food or water, it may do without.
Food	Place on lower surface or provide ramps for easy access. Raise the food bowl up by a couple inches, especially for arthritic cats. Food should be separate from water.
Water	Place on lower surface or provide ramps for easy access. Raise the water bowl up by a couple inches, especially for arthritic cats. Water should be separate from food.
Resting places	Provide multiple, elevated platforms with padded, comfortable bedding. Provide ramps for easy access. Warmed beds can be soothing.
Latrine sites	Provide 1 litter box per cat, plus 1 in multiple cat households. Use large, low-sided boxes for each access. Keep boxes within easy reach of the cats. Sandy-type litter is easier on cats' paws.
Hiding places or exit routes	Provide easily accessed hiding places, including elevated sites. Provide ramps for easy access. In multipet households, assure cats can have time alone if they desire. Do not presume an elderly cat can comfortably use a cat door flap.
Companionship	Elderly cats may have a decreased or increased desire for human companionship. Cat may grieve at the loss of a long-time companion. Introduction of a new cat or dog can be stressful for elderly cats.

issues. Dry, scaly skin may indicate poor nutrition or malabsorption or may suggest underlying disease. Likewise, changes in hair coat color, from black to brown, can be linked with malabsorption or deficiency of certain amino acids.

Changes in body weight (percent of prior weight), BCS, and muscle mass score (MMS) can be especially meaningful in older cats. Although BCS gives a good indication of body fat, MMS provides a better indication of lean muscle mass.[6,7] LBM decreases with age and with disease and can indicate underlying disease or malnutrition. Unintended weight loss should be evaluated further because it may be an indicator of chronic disease.

A nutritional assessment should be completed on aging patients. There are 3 parts to this assessment: (1) evaluation of the patient, (2) evaluation of the diet, and, (3) evaluation of the husbandry or feeding methodology. Detailed overviews regarding the nutritional assessment of cats and dogs have been published.[6,7] In addition, the World Small Animal Veterinary Association has developed several tools that can aid in nutritional assessment of patients that can be downloaded from the Web site: http://www.wsava.org/nutrition-toolkit.

Some key considerations regarding patients include life stage, lifestyle, body condition, and health. Increases or decreases in body condition or body weight should trigger further evaluation. A complete dietary evaluation must include everything that is consumed, including amounts of specific commercial foods, human foods, treats, and supplements. The nutritional characteristics of the total diet should be compared with an individual patient's needs. A diet may be complete and balanced yet be inappropriate for a specific patient. Feeding management evaluation assesses the amount and frequency fed as well as acceptance of food by a cat and any changes to a cat's appetite (representing ability and willingness to eat).

NUTRITIONAL REQUIREMENTS OF AGING CATS

Commercially available diets for senior cats can vary greatly in their nutrient content. For example, many senior cat diets are designed to be lower in calories to address the weight gain common in middle-aged cats. Such diets may not be suitable, however, for geriatric cats that have trouble maintaining their weight. Thus, dietary recommendations should consider a patient's individual needs.

Energy Requirements Change with Age

Aging cats, like dogs and humans, have a reduced energy requirement, and therefore a tendency for obesity.[1,8] This seems to be true for cats, however, only up to approximately 10 to 12 years of age.[8] Energy requirements increase beyond this point, especially after approximately 13 years of age.[4,9]

The increase in energy requirements may be due, at least in part, to a reduced digestive function in aging cats. A large percentage of aging cats have a reduced ability to digest fat: approximately 10% to 15% of mature cats and 33% of geriatric cats have reduced fat digestibility.[4] Although the onset of reduced digestive function may be gradual, in the long term it contributes negatively to the energy balance of a large number of geriatric cats. Reduced protein digestibility also occurs in geriatric cats.[4] One in 5 cats over the age of 14 years showed reduced ability to digest protein.[4] Reduced protein digestibility with age might contribute to negative nitrogen balance and loss of LBM.

Body Weight and Body Composition Changes with Age

Cats should be fed to maintain their optimal body weight. Long-term studies show that either obesity or excessive thinness increase mortality.[10] Although obesity itself contributes to reduced life span, it also increases the risk of many weight-related diseases, including diabetes mellitus, lameness (often due to arthritis), lower urinary tract diseases, liver disease (eg, hepatic lipidosis), and skin problems.[10–12]

On the other hand, many older cats experience weight loss and low body condition. This can result from several different, often interacting, factors. Weight loss despite normal to increased appetite may indicate hyperthyroidism (HT), diabetes mellitus, inflammatory bowel disease (IBD), or small cell intestinal lymphoma. Weight loss can be associated with inappetence and in older cats this may result from reduced senses of smell and taste and/or oral pain associated with periodontal disease. Dental disease, although common in older cats, is just one of many causes of poor appetite and weight loss. Reduced digestive function or altered metabolism also may contribute to weight loss.

Significant weight changes should always be investigated because weight loss is often the first sign of disease, as illustrated in a retrospective study of 258 cats.[4] In that study, cats that died of cancer, renal failure, or HT began losing weight approximately 2.25 years prior to death. Those dying from other causes began losing weight even earlier, at 3.75 years prior to death.

Concurrent with weight and fat loss, geriatric cats often experience age-associated loss of LBM, or sarcopenia. Even healthy geriatric cats have one-third less LBM compared with young adult cats.[4] The loss of LBM is even greater in many disease conditions. The loss of fat and muscle can contribute to the frail look of many geriatric patients and can contribute to reduced capacity for activity. Loss of LBM is a risk factor for mortality in humans and dogs and, apparently, also in cats.[13]

To help compensate for undesired loss of weight or condition, many older cats may benefit from a highly palatable, highly digestible, energy-dense food that is offered in small amounts frequently. Although not yet proved, prevention of weight loss in non-obese cats and maintenance of LBM may help delay morbidity and mortality. The limited research evidence currently available in cats is consistent with this: nonobese aging cats that were able to maintain fat and lean tissue mass lived longer than cats losing fat and LBM. In that study, preservation of body weight and body condition in nonobese cats had the strongest correlation with survival.[13] In addition to age, inadequate protein intake results in loss of LBM in adult cats.[14] Increased protein intake can help reduce, although not prevent, the age-associated loss of LBM.[15,16]

Balancing the Diet: Protein, Fat, and Carbohydrates

The ideal balance between dietary protein, fats, and carbohydrates is controversial and very much dependent on the needs of the individual cat.

Cats have a uniquely high requirement for dietary protein, which supports both protein turnover and continuous gluconeogenesis. When dietary protein intake is inadequate, cats (like other species) gradually deplete proteins in their LBM to support protein synthesis.[14] Traditional nitrogen balance studies indicate cats need less than 20% of their calories from protein. When maintenance of LBM is the defining criteria, however, adult cats require just over 5 g protein/kg body weight or approximately 34% of calories from protein.[14] For cats with low energy intake, a higher percentage from protein may be needed. For geriatric cats, this amount may increase further due to altered digestion and metabolism and age-related loss of LBM.[4,16]

Cats, like dogs, do not require a dietary source of carbohydrates. They have a physiologic requirement for carbohydrate (glucose) at the cellular level, however, and they are able to readily digest and use dietary carbohydrates.[17,18] When dietary carbohydrates are present, they can provide some or all of the cellular needs for glucose: when dietary carbohydrates are limited, the body produces glucose predominately from protein. Thus, dietary carbohydrates provide a protein-sparing effect.

In recent years, concern has been expressed about potential adverse effects of dietary carbohydrates in cats, specifically a proposed link between excess carbohydrate intake and diabetes or obesity.[19,20] There are few data, however, to support these concerns. Although some studies have shown a greater postprandial blood glucose concentration or alterations in glucose tolerance in cats after ingesting of high-carbohydrate, low-protein diets,[21–23] other studies have found no such effects,[17,24–27] indicating that components other than the amount of carbohydrate in the diet influence this effect. The feeding method (eg, single meal daily vs multiple meals or continuous access to food) also alters the glucose response with higher glucose peaks after a single large meal.[23,28,29] Furthermore, there is currently no evidence that the reported elevations in blood glucose or insulin are detrimental rather than simply physiologic. Published research also does not support a risk for obesity from carbohydrates in cat foods. On the contrary, multiple studies have shown that high-fat diets, rather than high-carbohydrate diets, increase the risk for obesity in cats.[10,30,31] Based on the relative risk for obesity, a preferred ratio of carbohydrate to fat in dry diets for adult cats has been proposed as a way to minimize undesired weight gain. For neutered cats, that ratio is 2 to 1 on an energy basis or approximately 4 times more carbohydrate than fat on an as-fed or dry matter basis.[32]

Minerals and vitamins must also be present in complete and balanced diets in appropriate amounts. Patients with subclinical disease associated with a mild malabsorption syndrome or polyuria may have increased losses of water-soluble nutrients, such as B vitamins, or fat-soluble nutrients, such as vitamins A and E. As discussed previously, many geriatric cats have a reduced ability to digest dietary fats. In these cats, absorption of several other essential nutrients, including B vitamins, vitamin E, potassium, and other minerals, was also compromised.[4] Geriatric cats with gastrointestinal disease are more likely to be deficient in cobalamin (vitamin B_{12}) compared with younger cats.[33,34] Thus, older cats should be carefully evaluated for possible nutrient deficiencies and may benefit from supplemental amounts of these nutrients.

Increased antioxidants may be beneficial for aging cats. Oxidative damage plays an important role in many diseases. Studies in dogs or cats have reported beneficial effects from increased amounts of dietary antioxidants on markers of oxidative status and are beginning to show benefits in certain disease states as well as for longevity.[35–38] In a study involving 90 aging cats, those fed a diet supplemented with vitamin E and β-carotene, a prebiotic, and essential fatty acids lived a full year longer than cats fed the basal diet without supplements.[37] Cats fed the basal diets supplemented only with vitamin E benefited but to a lesser degree.

Feeding Management

Feeding management addresses what, when, how, and where food is provided, and must meet the needs of both owner and patient. Feeding management also helps address some aspects of environmental enrichment and stress management, which can be particularly important in aging cats.

Some veterinarians recommend wet or canned food for aging cats to encourage water intake. When wet food is accepted by both cat and owner and added hydration is needed, this is a sensible approach. Some cats and some owners, however, prefer dry foods, and this also is completely acceptable. Specific diets should be recommended based on the energy and nutrient needs of a cat based on body condition, health, and metabolic needs. Cats, especially senior cats, should be fed on a set schedule. Some cats are stressed by unpredictable feeding times. When an owner is not able to accommodate a set schedule, automated feeders may be helpful.

Cats in multiple cat households may benefit from separate feeding bowls placed out of sight of each other. Bowls should be placed in quiet areas to keep cats from being disturbed while eating. Raised locations are desirable, as long as the aging cat can easily reach the feeding perch. Cats typically eat multiple small meals per day. Free access to food, however, removes any opportunity for cats to express their natural predatory instincts: failure to provide opportunities for predatory behavior may deprive cats of mental and physical activity.[39] Owners can address this by offering some or all of the daily food in puzzle or activity toys, such as food balls (**Fig. 1**) or other devices specifically designed to release food when played with by a cat. Food toys can be purchased from various sources and manufacturers or be homemade. Other options to encourage feeding-related activity include tossing kibbles for cats to chase or hiding food throughout the home.

Regardless of which diet is being fed, it is important to monitor intake to assure an appropriate amount of food is consumed. As discussed previously, mature cats have a high prevalence of obesity so avoiding excess intake is important. Geriatric cats, alternatively, have a tendency to lose weight. It is important to determine if weight loss is associated with normal, increased, or decreased food intake to help determine the cause. Reduced food intake in aging cats may be caused by dental disease in addition to metabolic and neurologic diseases. Pain from arthritis or associated inability to reach raised feeding platforms can also contribute to reduced intake. Cats under physical or emotional stress may respond with either increased or decreased intake. For example, food refusal is a common response to environmental threat.[39] Weight loss in the face of increased intake is suggestive of HT, diabetes mellitus, IBD, or small cell intestinal lymphoma.

If a dietary change becomes necessary, it is best to do so slowly. Provide both the old and new diets at the same time. One suggestion is to place the new food in the familiar feeding bowl and the familiar food in a new bowl, side by side. Allow the cat to become accustomed to the new food before slowly decreasing the amount of the prior diet. The transition may be accomplished in as little as 1 week in an otherwise healthy cat with a good appetite. For sick or inappetent cats or picky eaters, several weeks may be needed. Whenever possible, cats should be stable and eating well before introducing a new food to avoid the development of food aversion. It is best to avoid using the same food as the main meal to hide medications because this has the potential to create a food aversion. If medications need to be provided in food, one suggestion is to put it into a small amount of a different but palatable food, separate from the main meal.

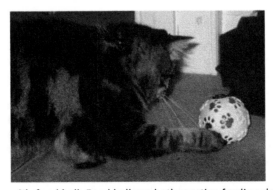

Fig. 1. Cat playing with food ball. Food balls and other active feeding devices can increase activity in cats.

THERAPEUTIC NUTRITION FOR SPECIFIC CONDITIONS
Feline Cognitive Dysfunction Syndrome

With increasing numbers of geriatric cats, there are more cats with signs of cognitive dysfunction syndrome (CDS).[40] Behavioral changes include excessive vocalization, inappropriate elimination, altered sleeping habits, and mood changes (irritability, restlessness, and disorientation).[41] Although CDS affects 28% to 50% of geriatric cats,[41,42] it is just one of several possible causes for behavioral changes in aging cats, so appropriate diagnostics must be performed.

Management of CDS involves environmental enrichment (leading to mental stimulation and increased activity) plus dietary management. Currently, there are few drugs or supplements with proved safety and efficacy in cats with CDS. In dogs and humans, antioxidants may reduce Alzheimer-like changes in brain function.[41,43] For example, feeding a diet enriched in antioxidants, L-carnitine, and omega-3 fatty acids plus providing environmental enrichment resulted in significant improvements in learning and memory in older dogs.[44,45] Medium-chain triglycerides are also proved to enhance brain function in dogs and humans.[46] A recent study in middle-aged and older cats found a combination of fish oil, antioxidants, arginine, and key B vitamins successfully enhanced brain functions.[42] A deficiency of these nutrients, especially omega-3 fatty acids and B vitamins, is a proved risk factor for brain aging, stroke, and dementia in humans. In another study, supplementing the diet of elderly cats with antioxidants, L-carnitine, docosahexaenoic acid, and sulfur amino acids resulted in increased activity compared with controls.[47]

There is a growing list of dietary supplements and compounds that may be beneficial for feline CDS,[41] including S-adenosylmethionine, which increases serotonin levels and has been shown to improve executive function in cats.[48] Placebo-controlled studies are needed, however, to see which may be beneficial, either as a single ingredient or in potentially synergistic combinations.

Unfortunately, once CDS is severe, instigating change can have a negative effect. Affected cats cope poorly to changes, whether diet, environment, or daily routine. Change should, therefore, be kept to a minimum and, when it cannot be avoided, made slowly and with reassurance.

Diabetes Mellitus

Diabetes mellitus is a complex disorder characterized by lack of insulin activity resulting in disturbances in glucose, lipid, and protein metabolism. A vast majority of diabetic cats have type 2 diabetes mellitus. The hallmarks of type 2 diabetes mellitus are decreased insulin secretion, especially in response to a glucose load, and insulin resistance.[49] Obesity and inactivity, both common in cats, seem to be significant risk factors for type 2 diabetes mellitus. In addition, glucose toxicity contributes to type 2 diabetes mellitus.[49] Correction of glucose toxicity can result in resolution of signs: up to 50% of cats newly diagnosed with diabetes may revert to a euglycemic state with careful management.[49,50]

Management involves insulin therapy coupled with appropriate dietary management. The focus of dietary management is to achieve and maintain ideal body condition and to help regulate glycemic control. Cats with type 2 diabetes mellitus may benefit from a high-protein (>45% dry basis), low-carbohydrate (<15% dry basis) (HPLC) diet as well as from eating small, frequent meals. The concept behind this is to minimize the postprandial glucose influx. Consumption of protein instead of soluble carbohydrates slows down absorption and release of glucose into the bloodstream. Consuming multiple small meals reduces the amount of glucose entering the bloodstream at any one time. Both of these help reduce the need for insulin.

Evidence to support the value of HPLC diets comes from multiple studies.[50–52] Many diabetic cats demonstrated decreased insulin requirements or enhanced glycemic control when fed an HPLC diet, and in many cases, insulin injections could be stopped altogether.[50–54] Because of the probability that insulin requirements decrease in cats fed HPLC diets, it is critical that these animals be carefully monitored to avoid hypoglycemia. Clients should be advised on what to look for and how to provide emergency care should a hypoglycemic crisis occur.

Obesity causes a reversible insulin resistance in tissues as a result of alterations in insulin receptor binding affinity and postreceptor defects that inhibit the movement of glucose into cells. When lean research cats were made obese by ad libitum feeding of high-fat diets, their insulin sensitivity decreased by 52%.[55] Even moderate increases in body weight can cause significant changes in insulin sensitivity, with a 30% decrease in insulin sensitivity for each kilogram increase in weight in adult cats.[24] Thus, prevention or correction of obesity should be attempted whenever possible.

Low-carbohydrate diets tend to be high in fat and calories. Therefore, for severely obese diabetic cats, it may be preferred to use a high-protein (>45% dry basis), high-fiber (5%–10% dry basis), moderate-carbohydrate (<25% dry basis) diet to facilitate weight loss. A few studies have evaluated fiber-supplemented diets for diabetic cats. Nelson and colleagues[56] reported a significant improvement in serum glucose concentrations in insulin-treated diabetic cats fed a diet containing 12% cellulose compared with a low-fiber diet. Two other studies reported a decrease in insulin requirements or improved glucose control in cats switched to a commercial high-fiber diet.[50,51] The benefits regarding glucose control were not as great with the high-fiber diets as from the HPLC diets, but they should enhance weight loss with significant long-term benefits.

Chronic Kidney Disease

The prevalence of chronic kidney disease (CKD) increases with age and affects as many as 10% of cats seen at university teaching hospitals.[57] More than 60% of these patients are 10 years of age or older. Although medical therapies, such as angiotensin-converting enzyme (ACE) inhibitors, calcium channel blockers, and so forth, continue to prove beneficial, dietary management remains an important factor in managing cats with CKD. Feeding cats with commercial diets formulated for cats with CKD resulted in longer survival with fewer uremic crises.[58,59] There remains controversy, however, as to which features of these diets are important and when to use them. Overall, the goals of dietary therapy are to provide patients with complete nutrition; to address the metabolic changes induced by disease, including clinical signs and consequences of uremic toxicity; and, if possible, to slow the progression of the disease. The International Renal Interest Society (IRIS) has proposed that management be determined based on the stage of the disease (www.iris-kidney.com) as well as on the presence of specific issues, such as hypertension, pyelonephritis, and nephroliths.[60]

There currently is no evidence of a benefit to dietary modification for patients before they reach IRIS stage 2 to 3. At that point, control of serum phosphorus, via restriction of dietary phosphorus and/or intestinal phosphate binders, is considered of prime importance.[60,61] Phosphorus intake or binders should be adjusted or added to maintain serum phosphorus concentrations within the low–normal range.

Diets supplemented with long-chain omega-3 fatty acids from fish oil may be beneficial from IRIS stage 2 onward. Cats showing proteinuria (urine protein/creatinine ratio of 0.2 or greater) at any stage of CKD may benefit from the protein restriction of typical renal diets as well as the higher levels of omega-3 fatty acids. ACE inhibitors, however, can be effective at reducing proteinuria and should be considered when a dietary change is contraindicated due to concurrent disease or other issues. Commercial renal diets are also formulated to address acid-base and electrolyte disorders that frequently occur in stage 3 to stage 4 CKD. Metabolic acidosis promotes many adverse clinical effects in renal patients, including anorexia, vomiting, lethargy, and weakness.[57] Salt restriction, once thought important for the management of hypertension, does not seem to be a significant factor in cats, and excessive sodium restriction is contraindicated.

Despite the importance of the factors discussed previously, the single biggest dietary adequacy factor is calorie intake. Weight loss with poor appetite is a common finding in cats with CKD.[57] Maintaining food intake and body weight is important to survival as well as preserving kidney function. It is always best to stabilize patients, regardless of illness, before attempting to change the diet to one that is fed long term. Cats should be introduced to the renal diet when they are at home and feeling well. Recommendations on introducing new diets are discussed previously. In advanced cases, feeding tubes can be used to improve nutritional status as well as hydration and to facilitate the administration of medications.

Osteoarthritis

Nutritional intervention can be beneficial for cats with osteoarthritis. Alterations involve weight loss in overweight cats, environmental changes to feeding stations, and, possibly, changes to the diet itself.

Reducing obesity reduces stress on a cat's joints, thereby reducing pain. Obesity management is addressed in greater detail in the article by Linder and Mueller elsewhere in this issue. Methods to encourage weight loss include giving less of a cat's normal diet, changing gradually to appropriate amounts of a weight-loss diet, and encouraging greater activity. Use of a feeding ball or food puzzle may be useful as long as a cat's arthritis does not prevent it from interacting with the device and obtaining its food. It is important to closely monitor a cat's weight because excessive or unintended weight loss may indicate that a cat no longer can gain access to its food, is experiencing food bowl competition in a multiple-cat household, or has developed significant systemic disease.

Aging and arthritic cats need easy access to all their key resources: food, water, litter box, resting places and hiding places, and exit routes. It is recommended that owners adjust their homes to accommodate their arthritic cats. This includes moving food and water bowls to lower surfaces or adding ramps to allow easier access to favored feeding stations and raising food and water bowls (**Fig. 2**). It is important to realize that although environmental changes help cats cope with arthritis and reduce the strain on joints, cats may still be in pain.

Although the evidence is limited for cats, it is suggested that some of the nutrient modifications that have proved helpful in other species, especially long-chain omega-3 fatty acids from fish oil, can also be of value in arthritic cats. A comprehensive review of published studies evaluating the use of nutraceuticals or diets to alleviate clinical signs of osteoarthritis, published in 2012, found only 1 peer-reviewed published study in cats.[62] That double-blind study evaluated a diet supplemented with fish oil, green-lipped mussel, glucosamine, and chondroitin sulfate, which resulted in a significant increase in activity in cats with moderate to severe osteoarthritis.[63] Another study, published to date only as an abstract, showed that a diet with added antioxidants (vitamins C and E and β-carotene), omega-3 fatty acids, chondroprotectants (methionine, glycosaminoglycans such as glucosamine and chondroitin sulfate), and L-carnitine and lysine (to aid obesity management and lean

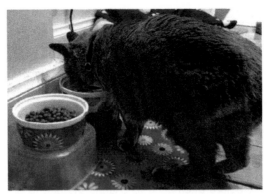

Fig. 2. Raised feeding bowl for cats with osteoarthritis. Raising the food and water bowls a couple of inches can make eating and drinking less painful for cats with arthritis of their front legs.

body mass) resulted in significant improvements versus the control diet when fed to older cats with osteoarthritis.[64]

Hyperthyroidism

HT is often described as a new condition that was rarely recognized in cats before 1979. Many reports, however, including a large study from Angell Animal Medical Center evaluating patients from 1949 to 1973, indicate that tumors of the feline thyroid were already common, especially in older cats.[65] At that time, less than 5% of feline patients were geriatric compared with 13% to 20% of cats in more recent reports.[1,2,65] In a new study of more than 400,000 cats, 0.9% were diagnosed with HT, and essentially 100% of these cats were greater than 10 years of age.[66] Thus, it seems that the current epidemic of HT may be the result of an older patient population combined with an increasing prevalence of diagnosis rather than a true increase in prevalence. Nevertheless, it seems a fairly common problem, especially in geriatric cats.

HT is one of many causes for aging cats to lose weight, but weight loss despite increased food intake should increase the suspicion of HT. After diagnosis, HT is primarily managed either medically or surgically. The role of diet, in most cases, is supportive. Many cats with HT have lost weight and LBM due to their disease. In addition, most are geriatric cats with increased protein requirements compared with younger cats.[16] Due to their hypermetabolic state, vitamin and other trace nutrient stores may be depleted. Insulin resistance and glucose intolerance are common problems in HT cats and seem to remain even after treatment.[67] To address these conditions, highly digestible, high-protein (>40% dry matter), low-carbohydrate (<25% dry matter) diets are recommended to help restore weight and LBM. Commercial kitten foods are a good option because they also provide increased amounts of vitamins and trace nutrients.

Recently, a diet restricted in iodine has been introduced as an alternative treatment of HT. The theory behind this diet is that it deprives the hyperactive thyroid tissue of iodine, which is essential for the production of thyroid hormones. Studies, published thus far only as abstracts, suggest that the low-iodine diets can reduce thyroxine levels to normal in HT cats,[68,69] making them a potential alternative to other therapeutic options as long as the diet is otherwise appropriate for a cat.

Although, to date, no side effects have been seen with the diet, iodine depletion is not without potential risk. Although the primary recognized role is for thyroid function, iodine also seems to play multiple other roles in the body. It serves as an antioxidant, promotes apoptosis, supports immune function, and may have antineoplastic bene-fits.[70,71] Chronic or early-life iodine deficiency predisposes to the development of HT when iodine sufficiency is subsequently restored.[72,73] Iodine-deficient diets pro-mote thyroid hypertrophy in cats as well as other species, and 1 epidemiologic study documented that cats consuming diets without added iodine had a 4-fold increased the risk for HT compared with those consuming diets with an iodine source.[74] Thus, it is not recommended to feed a low-iodine diet (eg, below maintenance requirements) to cats other than those with HT.

REFERENCES

1. Lund EM, Armstrong PJ, Kirk CA, et al. Health status and population character-istics of dogs and cats examined at private veterinary practices in the United States. J Am Vet Med Assoc 1999;214:1336–41.
2. Laflamme DP, Abood SK, Fascetti AJ, et al. Pet feeding practices among dog and cat owners in the United States and Australia. J Am Vet Med Assoc 2008;232:687–94.
3. Pittari J, Rodan I, Beekman G, et al. Senior care guidelines. American associa-tion of feline practitioners. J Feline Med Surg 2009;11:763–78.
4. Perez-Camargo G. Cat nutrition: what's new in the old? Comp Cont Edu Small Anim Pract 2004;26(Suppl 2A):5–10.
5. Fortney WD. Implementing a successful senior/geriatric health care program for veterinarians, veterinary technicians, and office managers. Vet Clin North Am Small Anim Pract 2012;42:823–34.
6. Baldwin K, Bartges J, Buffington T, et al. AAHA nutritional assessment guide-lines for dogs and cats. J Am Anim Hosp Assoc 2010;46:285–96.
7. Freeman L, Becvarova I, Cave N, et al. WSAVA nutritional assessment guide-lines. J Feline Med Surg 2011;13:516–25.
8. Laflamme DP, Ballam JM. Effect of age on maintenance energy requirements of adult cats [abstract]. Comp Cont Edu Small Anim Pract 2002;24(9A):82.
9. Cupp C, Perez-Camargo G, Patil A, et al. Long-term food consumption and body weight changes in a controlled population of geriatric cats [abstract]. Comp Cont Edu Small Anim Pract 2004;26(Suppl 2A):60.
10. Scarlett JM, Donoghue S. Associations between body condition and disease in cats. J Am Vet Med Assoc 1998;212:1725–31.
11. Scarlett JM, Donoghue S, Saidla J, et al. Overweight cats: perspectives and risk factors. Int J Obes 1994;18:S22–8.
12. Lund EM, Armstrong PJ, Kirk CA, et al. Prevalence and risk factors for obesity in adult cats from private US veterinary practices. Intern J Appl Res Vet Med 2005; 3:88–96.
13. Cupp CJ, Kerr WW. Effect of diet and body composition on life span in aging cats. Proc Nestle Purina Companion Animal Nutrition Summit: Focus on Geron-tology. Clearwater Beach (FL), March 26–7, 2010. p. 36–42.
14. Laflamme DP, Hannah SS. Discrepancy between use of lean body mass or ni-trogen balance to determine protein requirements for adult cats. J Feline Med Surg 2013;15:691–7.
15. Kealy RD. Factors influencing lean body mass in aging dogs. Comp Cont Edu Small Anim Pract 1999;21(11K):34–7.
16. Laflamme DP. Loss of lean body mass in aging cats is affected by age and diet. Eur Society Vet Comp Nutr Annual conference. Ghent (Belgium), September 19–21, 2013 [abstract].

17. Thiess S, Becskei C, Tomsa K, et al. Effects of high carbohydrate and high fat diet on plasma metabolite levels and on i.v. glucose tolerance test in intact and neutered male cats. J Feline Med Surg 2004;6:207–18.

18. de-Oliveira LD, Carciofi AC, Oliveira MC, et al. Effects of six carbohydrate sources on diet digestibility and postprandial glucose and insulin responses in cats. J Anim Sci 2008;86:2237–46.

19. Zoran DL. The carnivore connection to nutrition in cats. J Am Vet Med Assoc 2002;221:1559–67.

20. Rand JS, Fleeman LM, Farrow HE, et al. Canine and feline diabetes mellitus: nature or nurture? J Nutr 2004;134:2072S–80S.

21. Coradini M, Rand JS, Morton JM, et al. Effects of two commercially available feline diets on glucose and insulin concentrations, insulin sensitivity and energetic efficiency of weight gain. Br J Nutr 2011;106(Suppl 1):S64–77.

22. Hewson-Hughes AK, Gilham MS, Upton S, et al. The effect of dietary starch level on postprandial glucose and insulin concentrations in cats and dogs. Br J Nutr 2011;106:105S–9S.

23. Farrow HA, Rand JS, Morton JM, et al. Effect of dietary carbohydrate, fat and protein on postprandial glycemia and energy intake in cats. J Vet Intern Med 2013;27:1121–35.

24. Hoenig M, Thomaseth K, Waldron M, et al. Insulin sensitivity, fat distribution, and adipocytokine response to different diets in lean and obese cats before and after weight loss. Am J Physiol Regul Integr Comp Physiol 2007;292:R227–34.

25. Kley S, Hoenig M, Glushka J, et al. The impact of obesity, sex, and diet on hepatic glucose production in cats. Am J Physiol Regul Integr Comp Physiol 2009; 296:R936–43.

26. Martin LJM, Siliart B, Lutz TA, et al. Postprandial response of plasma insulin, amylin and acylated ghrelin to various test meals in lean and obese cats. Br J Nutr 2010;103:1610–9.

27. Hoenig M, Jordan ET, Glushka J, et al. Effect of macronutrients, age, and obesity on 6- and 24-h postprandial glucose metabolism in cats. Am J Physiol Regul Integr Comp Physiol 2011;301:R1798–807.

28. Brighenti F, Benini L, Del Rio D, et al. Colonic fermentation of indigestible carbohydrates contributes to the second-meal effect. Am J Clin Nutr 2006;83:817–22.

29. Hoenig M, Pach N, Thomaseth K, et al. Evaluation of long-term glucose homeostasis in lean and obese cats by use of continuous glucose monitoring. Am J Vet Res 2012;73:1100–6.

30. Nguyen PG, Dumon HJ, Siliart BS, et al. Effects of dietary fat and energy on body weight and composition after gonadectomy in cats. Am J Vet Res 2004; 65:1708–13.

31. Backus RC, Cave NJ, Keisler DH. Gonadectomy and high dietary fat but not high dietary carbohydrate induce gains in body weight and fat of domestic cats. Br J Nutr 2007;98:641–50.

32. Backus RC. Optimal and natural as rationale for selecting dietary energy distribution in carbohydrate and fat. Proc Nestle Purina Companion Animal Nutrition Summit. Atlanta (GA), March 21–23, 2013. p. 31–6.

33. Williams DA, Steiner JM, Ruaux CG. Older cats with gastrointestinal disease are more likely to be cobalamin deficient [abstract]. Comp Cont Edu Small Anim Pract 2004;26(Suppl 2A):62.

34. Simpson KW, Fyfe J, Cornetta A, et al. Subnormal concentrations of serum cobalamin (vitamin B12) in cats with gastrointestinal disease. J Vet Intern Med 2001;15:26–32.

35. Wedekind KJ, Zicker S, Lowry S, et al. Antioxidant status of adult beagles is affected by dietary antioxidant intake. J Nutr 2002;132:1658S–60S.
36. Brown SA. Oxidative stress and chronic kidney disease. Vet Clin North Am Small Anim Pract 2008;38:157–66.
37. Cupp CJ, Kerr WW, Jean-Philippe C, et al. The role of nutritional interventions in the longevity and maintenance of long-term health in aging cats. Intern J Appl Res Vet Med 2008;6:69–81.
38. Head E. Oxidative damage and cognitive dysfunction: antioxidant treatments to promote healthy brain aging. Neurchem Res 2009;34:670–8.
39. Herron M, Buffington CA. Environmental enrichment for indoor cats. Compend Contin Educ Vet 2010;32:E1–4.
40. Gunn-Moore DA. Cognitive dysfunction in cats: clinical assessment and management. Top Companion Anim Med 2011;26:17–24.
41. Landsberg G, Denenberg S, Araujo J. Cognitive dysfunction in cats: a syndrome we used to dismiss as "old age". J Feline Med Surg 2010;12:837–48.
42. Pan Y, Araujo JA, Burrows J, et al. Cognitive enhancement in middle-aged and old cats with dietary supplementation with a nutrient blend containing fish oil, B vitamins, antioxidants and arginine. Br J Nutr 2013;110:40–9.
43. Head E, Zicker SC. Nutraceuticals, aging and cognitive dysfunction. Vet Clin North Am Small Anim Pract 2004;34:217–28.
44. Milgram NW, Head E, Zicker SC, et al. Long-term treatment with antioxidants and a program of behavioral enrichment reduces age-dependent impairment in discrimination and reversal learning in beagle dogs. Exp Gerontol 2004;39: 753–65.
45. Milgram NW, Head E, Zicker SC, et al. Learning ability in aged beagle dogs is preserved by behavioural enrichment and dietary fortification: a two year longitudinal study. Neurobiol Aging 2005;26:77–90.
46. Pan Y, Larson B, Araujo JA, et al. Dietary supplementation with medium-chain TAG has long-lasting cognition-enhancing effects in aged dogs. Br J Nutr 2010;103:1746–54.
47. Houpt K, Levine E, Landsberg G, et al. Antioxidant fortified food improves owner perceived behaviour in aging the cat. Proceedings of the 2007 ESFM Conference. Prague (Czech Republic), 21–23, September, 2007.
48. Araujo JA, Faubert ML, Brooks ML, et al. NOVIFIT (NoviSAMe) tablets improve executive function in aged dogs and cats: implications for treatment of cognitive dysfunction syndrome. Intern J Appl Res Vet Med 2012;10:90–8.
49. Rand JS. Understanding feline diabetes. Comp Contin Educ Pract Vet 2002; 24(Suppl):2–6.
50. Bennett N, Greco DS, Peterson ME, et al. Comparison of a low carbohydrate-low fiber diet and a moderate carbohydrate-high fiber diet in the management of feline diabetes mellitus. J Feline Med Surg 2006;8:73–84.
51. Frank G, Anderson WH, Pazak HE, et al. Use of a high protein diet in the management of feline diabetes mellitus. Vet Ther 2001;2:238–46.
52. Mazzaferro EM, Greco DS, Turner SJ, et al. Treatment of feline diabetes mellitus using an alpha-glucosidase inhibitor and a low-carbohydrate diet. J Feline Med Surg 2003;5:183–9.
53. Marshall RD, Rand JS. Insulin glargine and a high protein-low carbohydrate diet are associated with high remission rates in newly diagnosed diabetic cats. J Vet Intern Med 2004;18:401 [abstr 63].
54. Rand JS, Marshall RD. Diabetes mellitus in cats. Vet Clin North Am Small Anim Pract 2005;35:211–24.

55. Appleton DJ, Rand JS, Sunvold GD. Insulin sensitivity decreases with obesity, and lean cats with low insulin sensitivity are at greatest risk of glucose intolerance with weight gain. J Feline Med Surg 2001;3:211–28.

56. Nelson RW, Scott-Moncrieff JC, Feldman EC, et al. Effect of dietary insoluble fiber on control of glycemia in cats with naturally acquired diabetes mellitus. J Am Vet Med Assoc 2000;216:1082–8.

57. Reynolds BS, Lefebvre HP, Feline CK. Pathophysiology and risk factors – what do we know? J Feline Med Surg 2013;15(Suppl 1):3–14.

58. Elliott J, Rawlings JM, Markwell PJ, et al. Survival of cat with naturally occurring chronic renal failure: effect of dietary management. J Small Anim Pract 2000;41: 235–42.

59. Ross SJ, Osborne CA, Kirk CA, et al. Clinical evaluation of dietary modification for treatment of spontaneous chronic kidney disease in cats. J Am Vet Med Assoc 2006;229:949–57.

60. Brown SA. Linking treatment to staging in chronic kidney disease. In: August JR, editor. Consultations in feline internal medicine, vol. 6. St Louis (MO): Saunders Elsevier; 2010. p. 475–82.

61. Kidder AC, Chew D. Treatment options for hyperphosphatemia in feline CKD: what's out there? J Feline Med Surg 2009;11:913–24.

62. Vandeweerd JM, Coisonon C, Clegg P, et al. Systematic review of efficacy of nutraceutical to alleviate clinical signs of osteoarthritis. J Vet Intern Med 2012;26: 448–56.

63. Lascelles BDX, DePuy V, Thomson A, et al. Evaluation of a therapeutic diet for feline degenerative joint disease. J Vet Intern Med 2010;24:487–95.

64. Fritsch D, Allen T, Sparkes A, et al. Improvement of clinical signs of osteoarthritis in cats by dietary intervention. Proc 18th ECVIM-CA Congress. Ghent (Belgium), September 4–6, 2008.

65. Leav I, Schiller AL, Rijnberk A, et al. Adenomas and carcinomas of the canine and feline thyroid. Am J Pathol 1976;83:61–122.

66. Klausner J. Banfield Pet Hospital state of pet health: 2012 report. Portland (OR): Banfield Pet Hospital; 2012.

67. Hoenig M, Peterson ME, Ferguson DC. Glucose tolerance and insulin secretion in spontaneously hyperthyroid cats. Res Vet Sci 1992;53:338–41.

68. Melendez LD, Yamka RM, Forrester SD, et al. Titration of dietary iodine for reducing serum thyroxine concentrations in newly diagnosed hyperthyroid cats [abstract]. J Vet Intern Med 2011;25:683.

69. Melendez LD, Yamka RM, Burris PA. Titration of dietary iodine for maintaining normal serum thyroxine concentrations in hyperthyroid cats [abstract]. J Vet Intern Med 2011;25:683.

70. Miller DW Jr. Extrathyroidal benefits of iodine. J Am Phys Surg 2006;11:106–10.

71. Aceves C, Anguiano B, Delgado G. The extrathyronine actions of iodine as antioxidant, apoptotic, and differentiation factor in various tissues. Thyroid 2013;23:938–46.

72. Speeckaert MM, Speeckaert R, Wierckx K, et al. Value and pitfalls in iodine fortification and supplementation in the 21st century. Br J Nutr 2011;106:964–73.

73. Van deVen A, Netea-Maier RT, Ross A, et al. Longitudinal trends in thyroid function in relation to iodine intake: ongoing changes of thyroid function despite adequate current iodine status. Eur J Endocrinol 2013;170:49–54. http://dx.doi.org/10.1530/EJE-13-0589.

74. Edinboro CH, Scott-Moncrieff JC, Glickman LT. Feline hyperthyroidism: potential relationship with iodine supplement requirements of commercial cat foods. J Feline Med Surg 2010;12:672–9.

Dietary Management of Feline Endocrine Disease

Mark E. Peterson, DVM[a,b,*], Laura Eirmann, DVM[c,d]

KEYWORDS

- Feline • Hyperthyroidism • Diabetes mellitus • Diet • Protein • Carbohydrate

KEY POINTS

- Hyperthyroidism is a hypermetabolic state that has profound effects on multiple organ systems (body condition, muscle, endocrine pancreas, parathyroid, and kidney).
- To best accomplish nutritional goals, hyperthyroid cats should be fed a diet containing a large amount of dietary protein (>40% of daily calories or metabolizable energy [ME] as protein; >12 g/100 kcal), a small amount of carbohydrate (<15% of total calories or ME; <4.5 g/100 kcal), and a moderate amount of phosphate (<250 mg of phosphate per 100 kcal).
- Dietary management plays a key role in the successful management of diabetic cats and should be used in conjunction with long-acting insulin treatment both to improve diabetic control and to help induce diabetic remission.
- Because cats are obligate carnivores, diabetic cats are carbohydrate intolerant and respond best to a low-carbohydrate diet (<12% ME; <3.5 g/100 kcal).
- Because diabetes is a catabolic state, weight loss, muscle wasting, and poor muscle condition scores are common in diabetic cats; therefore, feeding high-protein diets (>40% ME; >12 g/100 kcal) is recommended to help maintain muscle mass.

INTRODUCTION

When treating cats with endocrine disease, most veterinarians concentrate on medical or surgical treatments that can be used to manage or cure the disease. Dietary issues are frequently ignored or not properly addressed. However, nutritional support can play an integral role in the successful management of feline endocrine diseases.

This article discusses the 2 most common endocrine problems of cats seen in clinical practice (ie, hyperthyroidism and diabetes mellitus) and discusses the way

Funding sources: None.
Conflict of interest: None (M.E. Peterson); Veterinary Communications Manager, Nestle Purina PetCare (L. Eirmann).
[a] Animal Endocrine Clinic, 21 West 100th Street, New York, NY 10025, USA; [b] Department of Clinical Sciences, New York State College of Veterinary Medicine, Cornell University, Ithaca, New York 14853, USA; [c] Oradell Animal Hospital, 580 Winters Avenue, Paramus, NJ 07652, USA; [d] Nestle Purina PetCare, St Louis, MO 63102, USA
* Corresponding author.
E-mail address: drpeterson@animalendocrine.com

nutrition can be integrated into the management of these common feline diseases. The goal is to use the cat's diet as a means to support its overall body health and metabolism and, therefore, help manage its underlying endocrine disease.

HYPERTHYROIDISM IN CATS

Hyperthyroidism is the most common endocrine disorder of cats, and is one of the most common medical problems seen in small animal practice, affecting approximately 10% of all senior and geriatric cats more than 10 years of age.[1–3] Despite nutritional factors and cat food having been proposed to have a role in the etiopathogenesis of this disease,[4,5] there are only limited published recommendations about what to feed these cats. The question of what to feed a hyperthyroid cat is commonly asked by concerned cat owners.

The Many Metabolic Problems Facing the Hyperthyroid Cat

When secreted in excess, thyroid hormones have profound metabolic effects on the body, and dysfunction of multiple organ systems (central nervous, cardiac, gastrointestinal, hepatic, pancreatic, and renal systems) is common in hyperthyroid cats.[1–3,6]

Weight loss and muscle wasting

Despite a normal to increased appetite, weight loss is the classic and most common sign seen in cats with hyperthyroidism.[1–3,6] These cats lose weight because their hyperthyroidism accelerates their metabolic rate such that energy demand exceeds energy consumption. It is important to realize that hyperthyroidism is a catabolic state.[7,8] The progressive weight loss and muscle wasting that is so characteristic of feline hyperthyroid disease is caused by increased protein catabolism leading to a negative nitrogen balance.[9–11]

When hyperthyroid cats first lose weight, the disorder can usually be first noticed as a loss of muscle mass in the cat's lumbar paravertebral area. Despite this loss of muscle mass, most mildly hyperthyroid cats retain their abdominal adipose tissue during the initial stages of their thyroid disease and may even have a higher than ideal body condition score (BCS). With time, severe muscle wasting, emaciation, cachexia, and death from starvation can occur if the cat's hyperthyroidism is left untreated.[1,2]

In hyperthyroidism, the cat's body consumes its own muscle tissue to meet its protein needs. Even with treatment of hyperthyroidism, recovery of muscle mass and function may be prolonged, lasting several weeks to months.[9] This is especially true if these cats are not provided with enough dietary protein to help rebuild their lost muscle mass.[12]

Hyperglycemia, glucose intolerance, insulin resistance, and overt diabetes

In both humans and experimental animals, thyroid hormone excess affects many aspects of metabolism and energy homeostasis, including the development of glucose intolerance and insulin resistance.[13,14] Hyperthyroid cats also develop changes in glucose and insulin metabolism. Mild to moderate hyperglycemia is common in hyperthyroid cats, which is generally attributed to a stress reaction.[1–3] However, the underlying metabolic changes reported in hyperthyroid cats are more complicated: hyperthyroidism frequently causes moderate to severe endogenous insulin resistance, as shown by high resting serum insulin concentrations and an exaggerated insulin response during an intravenous glucose tolerance test.[15,16] This insulin resistance is associated with a decreased glucose clearance (impaired glucose tolerance), which indicates a prediabetic state.

Untreated hyperthyroid cats sometimes develop overt diabetes mellitus.[17,18] Many of these diabetic cats develop moderate resistance to the injected insulin, with poor diabetic control.[17,19] However, the insulin resistance and prediabetic state that is so common in hyperthyroid cats does not always improve and may even worsen despite successful treatment of hyperthyroidism,[16,17] which indicates that hyperthyroid cats may have long-lasting alterations of glucose tolerance and insulin secretion that cannot always be reversed by correction of the hyperthyroid state. Some of these hyperthyroid cats (not diabetic at time of diagnosis) go on to develop overt diabetes mellitus in the months to years after treatment of hyperthyroidism. Most cats that develop diabetes after the hyperthyroid state has been corrected have become overweight or obese, which may also contribute to the development of their diabetes.[20]

Hyperphosphatemia, secondary hyperparathyroidism, and chronic kidney disease

Hyperthyroidism and chronic kidney disease (CKD) are both common disorders in senior and geriatric cats. Therefore, both disorders frequently develop together in the same cat. The prevalence of CKD in the geriatric cat population has variably been reported as 7.7% of cats more than 10 years of age,[21] 15.3% of geriatric cats more than 15 years of age,[22] and 30% of geriatric cats more than 15 years of age.[23] By comparison, the prevalence of CKD in hyperthyroid cats (average age of 12–13 years) has been reported as 30% to 40%.[2,24–27] The higher-than-expected prevalence of CKD in hyperthyroid cats suggests that thyrotoxicosis may contribute to the development or progression of CKD in cats.

Hyperthyroidism could damage the feline kidney by several mechanisms. In the hyperthyroid state, volume expansion occurs secondary to activation of the renin-angiotensin-aldosterone system.[25,28] There is also sympathetic activation, leading to an increase in the heart rate.[1–3,25] Both of these alterations tend to increase the renal blood flow and the glomerular filtration rate (GFR), and could lead to glomerular hypertension.[24–27] When the GFR is increased in a hyperthyroid cat with underlying CKD, it can mask renal insufficiency; serum concentrations of urea nitrogen and creatinine may be normal despite mild to moderate kidney disease. Decreased muscle mass, which is a common feature of hyperthyroidism, also contributes to the reduced serum creatinine concentration in these cats (because creatinine is derived from muscle tissue).[1–3,24–27]

Successful treatment of hyperthyroidism restores the high serum T_4 concentration to normal and, in cats without CKD, also returns the high GFR back to euthyroid values. However, in cats with CKD, the GFR decreases to the low-normal or subnormal levels expected with moderate renal dysfunction.[24–27] Therefore, this decrease in GFR can result in the worsening of the serum kidney function tests. In these cases, although the CKD was present before treatment, the kidney disease was masked by the hyperdynamic state of the hyperthyroidism.[24,25]

In addition to the hyperthyroid-induced increase in renal hemodynamics, hyperthyroid cats may develop several metabolic disturbances that may contribute to progression of renal disease. Between a third to half of hyperthyroid cats develop hyperphosphatemia,[29–31] and about 60% of hyperthyroid cats have high plasma concentrations of parathyroid hormone (PTH).[27,30,32] This combination of hyperphosphatemia and high PTH concentrations is consistent with secondary renal hyperparathyroidism, which could indicate the presence of underlying kidney disease in these cats.[33,34] Because PTH is classified as a uremic toxin, such hyperthyroid-associated increases in plasma PTH concentrations could be a mechanism of renal damage leading to increased morbidity and mortality in cats with hyperthyroidism.

Sarcopenia of aging

In addition to loss of muscle mass from the catabolic effects of thyroid hormone excess, cats also tend to lose muscle mass as they age, independent of their thyroid status. This phenomenon, referred to as sarcopenia of aging, is also common in elderly people.[35,36] The term age-related sarcopenia is derived from Greek (meaning poverty of flesh) and is characterized by a degenerative loss of skeletal muscle mass and strength, as well as increased muscle fatigability.[37,38]

In adult cats, maintenance energy requirements decrease by about 3% per year until the age of 11 years, and then start to increase again.[39] This process contributes to a tendency of senior and geriatric cats to lose weight if their energy needs are not met. Lean body mass of aging cats decreases dramatically after 12 years of age, and by age 15 years, cats may have lean tissue mass (ie, muscle) that is a third less than cats aged 7 years or less.[40,41] Body fat also tends to progressively decrease in cats after the age of 12 years; this combination of reduced lean mass and body fat contributes to the weight loss experienced by many elderly cats.

The ability to digest protein is also compromised in many geriatric cats. After the age of 14 years, one-fifth of geriatric cats have reduced ability to digest protein.[39-41] Reduced protein digestibility in geriatric cats seems to occur in parallel with reduction of lean tissue, and it might predispose them to negative nitrogen balance.[42]

Recent studies of both adult and senior cats indicate that the daily protein requirements of adult cats needed to maintain lean body mass (≈ 5 g/kg body weight) is considerably higher than that currently recommended for adult maintenance by either the Association of American Feed Control Officials (AAFCO) or National Research Council (NRC) guidelines.[43,44] Feeding a higher protein, highly digestible, energy-dense diet to senior and geriatric cats may prevent or slow their decline in body weight and lean body tissue associated with aging.[39,42,45] Limiting protein intake in geriatric cats, at a time when lean tissue has been lost, only hastens the progression of muscle wasting.

Because more than 95% of all cats with hyperthyroidism are more than 10 years of age,[1,2] almost all hyperthyroid cats can be considered to be a senior or geriatric.[46] Therefore, sarcopenia of aging contribute to the loss of lean body mass induced by the catabolic effect of chronic hyperthyroidism, even after the cat's hyperthyroid state has been successfully treated.

Management Goals

Hyperthyroidism in cats is best treated medically, with chronic administration of an antithyroid drug to block thyroid hormone secretion, with surgical thyroidectomy to remove the affected thyroid adenoma(s), or with radioiodine to irradiate and destroy the thyroid adenoma(s).

The adjunctive goals of nutritional management of cats with hyperthyroidism are to provide a diet that allows weight gain (back to optimal body weight) and helps restore loss of muscle mass; a diet that lessens postprandial hyperglycemia, improves insulin sensitivity, and helps stabilize glucose metabolism; and a diet that helps control hyperphosphatemia and secondary hyperparathyroidism and slows the progression of any underlying kidney disease.

Nutritional Strategies and Recommendations for Hyperthyroid Cats

High dietary protein

Obligate carnivores, such as the cat, are unique in their need for large amounts of dietary protein (specifically, dispensable nitrogen), which distinguishes them from omnivores and herbivore species.[47-49] This absolute requirement for dietary protein intake in cats is critically important when formulating a diet for hyperthyroid cats, in which protein catabolism and muscle wasting is universally present.

Assuming adequate calorie intake, protein is the primary macronutrient responsible for maintenance of muscle mass.[38] Restoring and preserving remaining muscle tissue in cats treated for hyperthyroidism depends on the cat consuming a diet with sufficient amounts of high-quality protein. We recommend a target of 40% or more of daily calories from protein, or greater than or equal to 12 g/100 kcal metabolizable energy (ME).

This recommendation for larger amounts of dietary protein does not change once euthyroidism has been restored. The dogma that all senior and geriatric cats should be fed reduced-energy senior diets must be questioned based on what is now known about the increasing energy requirements and nutritional needs of these cats.[36,39–45] In most senior and geriatric cats,[46] logic dictates the use of highly digestible, energy-dense food to mitigate the decline in body weight and lean body tissue and to avoid protein/calorie malnutrition.[36,42,45] Reducing protein intake in geriatric cats, at a time when lean tissue has been lost, is contraindicated; when deprived of adequate amounts of dietary protein, carnivores continue to break down muscle tissue to support protein turnover.[47,48] Feeding larger amounts of high-quality protein can help to restore and maintain lost muscle mass in these cats, because many develop sarcopenia as they age.

Low dietary carbohydrates

Because most of these cats also have subclinical diabetes, as shown by their mild hyperglycemia, glucose intolerance, and insulin resistance,[15,16] feeding a low-carbohydrate diet is also strongly recommended. To this end, we recommend a target of less than 15% of total calories from carbohydrates, or less than 4.5 g/100 kcal ME. Feeding a low-carbohydrate diet lessens postprandial hyperglycemia, improves insulin sensitivity, reduces the potential need for exogenous insulin, and helps stabilize glucose metabolism in these cats with subclinical diabetes,[50–54] and may prevent the development of overt diabetes after successful control of the hyperthyroidism.

Low-carbohydrate diets must contain moderate to large amounts of fat (eg, if 10% of calories are fed as carbohydrate and 40% of calories as protein, the remaining 50% of calories must come from fat). For the underweight hyperthyroid cat, this caloric density of fat can be advantageous. However, after the hyperthyroidism is controlled, caloric intake, body weight, and BCS must be monitored to ensure that the cat does not become overweight or obese, which would also predispose to diabetes.[20]

Lower dietary phosphate

If concurrent CKD is documented, either before or after treatment of hyperthyroidism, mild to moderate reduction of dietary phosphate is recommended, depending on the severity of the CKD. Secondary renal hyperparathyroidism may contribute to the progression of CKD in cats, and the feeding of phosphate-restricted diets to cats with CKD can reduce PTH concentrations in cats with CKD[33,55] and improve survival time.[34,56,57]

We determine the severity of the cat's CKD by use of the International Renal Interest Society (IRIS) staging system, which is based on the plasma creatinine concentration (ie, stage 1, <1.6 mg/dL; stage 2, 1.6–2.8 mg/dL; stage 3, 2.9–5.0 mg/dL; and stage 4, >5 mg/dL).[58]

The phosphate content in adult feline maintenance diets can encompass a wide range, from diets that contain phosphate levels only just more than the AAFCO minimum (125 mg/100 kcal[59]) to levels of more than 500 mg/100 kcal. In cats with mild CKD (IRIS stage 1 or 2), we recommend feeding a diet containing a phosphate content at the lower end of this range (eg, 125–250 mg of phosphate per 100 kcal), adjusted as needed to maintain serum phosphate concentrations within the IRIS target range for cats with CKD (ie, 2.5–4.5 mg/dL).[57,60] In some cats, dietary phosphate may need to be further restricted to less than 125 mg/100 kcal to achieve the target serum phosphate concentrations. Again, because a lower phosphate diet that also contains large amounts of protein and small amounts of carbohydrates is ideal, most over-the-counter diets do not meet all of these criteria. Information concerning the phosphate concentrations of cat foods is available from the company's product guide or by calling the pet food company.

For hyperthyroid cats with more advanced CKD (IRIS stage 3–4), phosphate restriction to levels less than the AAFCO minimum may be indicated.[55,56] For this purpose, feeding a phosphate-restricted diet (<125 mg per 100 kcal) is recommended. This intake can most easily be accomplished by feeding a prescription kidney diet; however, none of these commercial kidney diets meets our other recommendations for higher protein (>40% ME; >12 g/100 kcal) and lower carbohydrate (<15% ME; <4.5 g/100 kcal) levels in these senior and geriatric cats. As an alternative, a high-protein, low-carbohydrate diet can be formulated that is also low in phosphorus. Other supplements to consider in these cats, which are routinely added to prescription kidney diets, include omega-3 fatty acids, potassium gluconate, and water-soluble B-complex vitamins.[55,56]

If a low-phosphate diet cannot be fed or serum phosphate concentrations remain above the target concentration recommended by IRIS for the specific stage of CKD, the use of phosphate binders is needed.[55] Aluminum hydroxide (100 mg/kg/d) is commonly used and can be mixed with canned or dry food.

DIABETES MELLITUS

Diet plays a key role in the successful management of the diabetic cat. However, the principles for management of diabetes mellitus differ greatly between dogs and cats with this disorder. Unlike canine diabetes, which results from absolute insulin deficiency secondary to beta-cell destruction (similar to type I diabetes in humans), feline diabetes is generally classified as type 2, characterized by insulin resistance and glucose intolerance but with some residual capacity to produce insulin. In diabetic dogs, lifelong exogenous insulin is the mainstay of therapy and remission of diabetes is not expected, whereas remission of diabetes is possible in cats.[50,51,54]

Dietary therapy is of utmost importance in the successful management of diabetic cats and should be used in conjunction with long-acting insulin treatment both to improve diabetic control and to help induce diabetic remission. Diabetic cats are carbohydrate intolerant and respond best to a low-carbohydrate diet; this again differs from dogs, which are omnivores and are more tolerant of a meal that is moderate to high in carbohydrates, even when diabetic.[61]

Of comparative interest, especially for feline diabetes, is the realization that carbohydrate-restriction was the only successful treatment of human diabetic patients in the preinsulin era.[62,63] After the introduction of insulin in 1922 and oral hypoglycemic medications in 1942,[63] the dietary recommendations changed to include more carbohydrate intake because most experts reasoned that the medications would keep the blood glucose concentrations in control. Over the last decade, the recommendations have gradually changed, with many diabetologists again recommending lower carbohydrate diets for their patients with type 2 diabetes, because this is a disorder of carbohydrate intolerance.[64–68] One of the main advantages of carbohydrate restriction is that it allows control of hyperglycemia with lower doses of insulin, thus lessening the risk of hypoglycemia.[69] Similar findings are reported in diabetic cats with type 2 diabetes managed with a low-carbohydrate diet.[51,54]

The Many Metabolic Problems Facing the Diabetic Cat

Diabetes mellitus can be associated with profound metabolic effects on the whole body, leading to hyperglycemia, ketosis, hyperlipidemia, azotemia, and electrolyte imbalances. Dysfunction of multiple organ systems (pancreatic, hepatic, renal, and peripheral nervous systems) is common in cats with diabetes mellitus.[50,70] Like hyperthyroidism, uncontrolled diabetes is a catabolic condition, so although obesity predisposes the cat to becoming diabetic, loss of weight, and especially loss of lean body mass, is common in cats with diabetes.

Hyperglycemia, insulin resistance, decreased insulin secretion, glucose toxicity

Based on clinical characteristics and islet pathology, approximately 90% of diabetic cats seem to have type 2 diabetes mellitus, which results from a combination of impaired insulin secretion, insulin resistance, and amyloid deposition in the pancreatic islets.[20] Insulin resistance is a hallmark of type 2 diabetes. Diabetic cats are, on average, 6 times less sensitive to insulin than are healthy cats.[70] Weight gain and obesity, which are common in cats that become diabetes, has a particularly profound effect on insulin resistance.

Loss of beta-cell function is another hallmark of type 2 diabetes mellitus.[20] The mechanisms of beta-cell failure are still debated, but intracellular amyloid oligomers are a likely contributor in early stages.[20,71] Insulin resistance and glucose toxicity further contribute to beta-cell damage and maintenance of the diabetic state.[20,72,73] Glucose toxicity describes the phenomenon of suppression of insulin secretion from beta cells secondary to prolonged hyperglycemia.[20,70,73] Glucose toxicity is dose dependent, with greater suppression occurring with more severe hyperglycemia. Suppression of insulin secretion by glucose toxicity is initially reversible but eventually results in the irreversible loss of beta cells.[20,72,73] This process explains why cats with poorly controlled diabetes for longer than 6 months have a reduced probability of remission, even after good glycemic control is achieved.

Weight loss or gain, obesity, muscle wasting

At the time of diabetes diagnosis, weight loss is reported in about 70% of cats.[74] However, cats are more often overweight or obese (40%) than of normal weight or underweight.[70,74] Muscle wasting and poor muscle condition scores are detected in about half of cats with diabetes.[70,74]

Sarcopenia of aging

Epidemiologic studies in cats consistently show diabetes to be a disease of senior cats. Like cats with hyperthyroidism, the typical diabetic cat is a senior, with about 70% more than 10 years of age at time of diagnosis.[50,70] Therefore, because most of these cats are senior, they are also prone to develop sarcopenia of aging, as discussed earlier.

In human patients, type 2 diabetes is associated with an increased risk of concurrent sarcopenia.[75] In addition, because skeletal muscle is a primary site for insulin-mediated glucose uptake and deposition, sarcopenia (and especially sarcopenic obesity[76]) may promote insulin resistance, predisposing to the development of type 2 diabetes and making diabetes more resistant to control.[77,78]

It is not known whether the loss of muscle mass alone (sarcopenia) or combined with weight gain (sarcopenic obesity), which are both commonly seen in cats with diabetes, also contributes to the insulin resistance and hyperglycemia associated with the feline disorder. However, it is reasonable to assume that sarcopenia and sarcopenic obesity may do so in cats, as they do in humans.

Nutritional Management Goals

In cats with diabetes, a primary goal of dietary therapy is to feed a diet that lessens postprandial hyperglycemia, reduces marked fluctuations of blood glucose concentrations, minimizes the demand on beta cells to produce insulin, and improves insulin sensitivity. By doing this, the effect of glucose toxicity is decreased and it is hoped that the pancreatic islet cells are allowed to recover, leading to remission of the diabetic state.[20,70,73] A secondary goal of therapy is to provide a diet that helps to normalize body weight and maintain and/or restore lost muscle mass.

Nutritional Strategies and Recommendations for Diabetic Cats

Low dietary carbohydrates

As recommended in recent diabetes management guidelines,[51] most practicing veterinarians who specialize in feline medicine agree that feeding a low-carbohydrate diet is a mainstay in the treatment of diabetes mellitus, especially if remission of the diabetic state is the goal. In accord with that, there is strong clinical and research evidence that a diet containing low concentrations of carbohydrate (eg, carbohydrates <12% of calories or ME; <3.5 g/100 kcal) is an effective means for achieving nutritional goals for cats with diabetes.[51,54,79-84] Feeding a high-protein, low-carbohydrate diet improves insulin sensitivity, helps stabilize glucose metabolism, and can reduce or eliminate the need for exogenous insulin in many cats, especially if also treated with an intensive insulin regimen.[51,54,79-85] The likely mechanism for these observations is simple: decreasing dietary carbohydrate load reduces the postprandial blood glucose increase, which in diabetic cats can be prolonged, sometimes lasting for more than 12 hours.

If a change in feeding to a low-carbohydrate diet is made in a diabetic cat already stabilized on insulin, it is likely to result in a reduced daily insulin requirement (often significantly reduced).[54,70] If not closely monitored, ideally with home glucose testing, severe hypoglycemia can develop in these cats. Therefore, when changing from a high-carbohydrate to a low-carbohydrate diet, we recommend initially reducing the insulin dose by 30% to 50% to help avoid hypoglycemia.

If the diabetic cat goes into remission (no more insulin needed to maintain euglycemia), we recommend maintaining the low-carbohydrate diet for life to help prevent or delay relapse of the diabetic state.

High dietary protein

Because diabetes is a catabolic state, loss of muscle mass is common in cats with diabetes, even if their BCS indicates overweight or obesity. In these cats, it is essential to feed a diet containing adequate amounts of protein to ensure maintenance of lean body mass in this catabolic diabetic state. Feeding a higher protein diet might also help restore some of the lost muscle mass in these cats, once insulin therapy is instituted. In addition, higher protein diets help prevent hepatic lipidosis from developing during induction of weight loss (needed in many diabetic cats), and are essential to increasing metabolism to help promote fat burning and normal insulin function.[54,86,87] In addition, the higher fed protein is used to provide needed glucose in cats fed a low-carbohydrate diet; however, because this endogenously produced glucose is released into the bloodstream slowly, this helps maintain a euglycemic balance in the diabetic cat.

Protein is the primary macronutrient responsible for maintenance of muscle mass.[38,42] Restoring and preserving remaining muscle tissue in diabetic cats, an obligate carnivore, depends on the cat consuming a diet with sufficient amounts of high-quality protein. We recommend diets that provide at least 40% of calories as protein (>12 g/100 kcal).[51] This higher-than-average protein level also helps restore and maintain lost muscle mass, because many diabetic cats develop sarcopenia as they age.

Although it is important to implement a low-carbohydrate/high-protein diet in the management of most cats with diabetes as soon as possible, there are circumstances in which this should be delayed or may be inappropriate.[54] For example, in cats with advanced (IRIS stage 3–4) CKD requiring phosphorus restriction and a reduction in dietary protein, high-protein/low-carbohydrate diabetic diets may not be appropriate. In cats with earlier stages of CKD, phosphorus should be restricted, if possible using methods other than changing to a protein-restricted diet (higher in carbohydrate), because this is likely to reduce the probability of remission. In cats with later stages of CKD or in those cats in which remission is unlikely, use of a prescription kidney diet is recommended. Over-the-counter low-carbohydrate cat foods may have substantially higher phosphate levels than some of the veterinary therapeutic diets designed for diabetes. Therefore, the nutrient profile of the specific product must be obtained to determine whether the product meets the desired nutrient goals for that patient.

Low-carbohydrate diets contain moderate to large amounts of fat (eg, if 12% of calories are fed as carbohydrate and 45% of calories as protein, the remaining 43% of calories must come from fat). For the underweight diabetic cat, this caloric density of fat can be advantageous. However, in the overweight diabetic cat or in the controlled normal-weight diabetic, caloric intake, body weight, and BCS must be monitored to ensure that the cat does not become overweight or obese, which would also worsen insulin resistance and may lead to relapse of diabetes in those cats placed into remission.[20]

REFERENCES

1. Baral RM, Peterson ME. Thyroid gland disorders: hyperthyroidism and hypothyroidism. In: Little SE, editor. The cat: clinical medicine and management. St Louis (MO): Elsevier Saunders; 2012. p. 571–92.
2. Mooney CT, Peterson ME. Feline hyperthyroidism. In: Mooney CT, Peterson ME, editors. BSAVA manual of canine and feline endocrinology. 4th edition. Quedgeley (United Kingdom): British Small Animal Veterinary Association; 2012. p. 92–110.
3. Peterson ME. Hyperthyroidism in cats. In: Rand JS, Behrend E, Gunn-Moore D, et al, editors. Clinical endocrinology of companion animals. Ames (Iowa): Wiley-Blackwell; 2013. p. 295–310.
4. Peterson ME, Ward CR. Etiopathologic findings of hyperthyroidism in cats. Vet Clin North Am Small Anim Pract 2007;37:633–45, v. Available at: http://www.ncbi.nlm.nih.gov/pubmed/17619003.
5. Peterson M. Hyperthyroidism in cats: what's causing this epidemic of thyroid disease and can we prevent it? J Feline Med Surg 2012;14:804–18. Available at: http://www.ncbi.nlm.nih.gov/pubmed/23087006.
6. Peterson ME, Kintzer PP, Cavanagh PG, et al. Feline hyperthyroidism: pretreatment clinical and laboratory evaluation of 131 cases. J Am Vet Med Assoc 1983; 183:103–10. Available at: http://www.ncbi.nlm.nih.gov/pubmed/6874510.
7. Kekki M. Serum protein turnover in experimental hypo- and hyperthyroidism. Acta Endocrinol (Copenh) 1964;46(Suppl 91):91–137. Available at: http://www.ncbi.nlm.nih.gov/pubmed/14186609.
8. Hamwi GJ, Tzagournis M. Nutrition and diseases of the endocrine glands. Am J Clin Nutr 1970;23:311–29. Available at: http://www.ncbi.nlm.nih.gov/pubmed/4908257.
9. Norrelund H, Hove KY, Brems-Dalgaard E, et al. Muscle mass and function in thyrotoxic patients before and during medical treatment. Clin Endocrinol (Oxf) 1999;51:693–9. Available at: http://www.ncbi.nlm.nih.gov/pubmed/10619973.

10. Riis AL, Jorgensen JO, Gjedde S, et al. Whole body and forearm substrate metabolism in hyperthyroidism: evidence of increased basal muscle protein breakdown. Am J Physiol Endocrinol Metab 2005;288:E1067–73. Available at: http://www.ncbi.nlm.nih.gov/pubmed/15657093.

11. Riis AL, Jorgensen JO, Ivarsen P, et al. Increased protein turnover and proteolysis is an early and primary feature of short-term experimental hyperthyroidism in healthy women. J Clin Endocrinol Metab 2008;93:3999–4005. Available at: http://www.ncbi.nlm.nih.gov/pubmed/18628521.

12. Freeman LM. Cachexia and sarcopenia: emerging syndromes of importance in dogs and cats. J Vet Intern Med 2012;26:3–17. Available at: http://www.ncbi.nlm.nih.gov/pubmed/22111652.

13. Mitrou P, Raptis SA, Dimitriadis G. Insulin action in hyperthyroidism: a focus on muscle and adipose tissue. Endocr Rev 2010;31:663–79. Available at: http://www.ncbi.nlm.nih.gov/pubmed/20519325.

14. Raboudi N, Arem R, Jones RH, et al. Fasting and postabsorptive hepatic glucose and insulin metabolism in hyperthyroidism. Am J Physiol 1989;256:E159–66. Available at: http://www.ncbi.nlm.nih.gov/pubmed/2643338.

15. Hoenig M, Ferguson DC. Impairment of glucose tolerance in hyperthyroid cats. J Endocrinol 1989;121:249–51. Available at: http://www.ncbi.nlm.nih.gov/pubmed/2666555.

16. Hoenig M, Peterson ME, Ferguson DC. Glucose tolerance and insulin secretion in spontaneously hyperthyroid cats. Res Vet Sci 1992;53:338–41. Available at: http://www.ncbi.nlm.nih.gov/pubmed/1465507.

17. Peterson ME. The difficult diabetic: Acromegaly, Cushing's, and other causes of insulin resistance. Small Animal & Exotics Proceedings, Vol. 26. Gainesville (FL): North American Veterinary Conference (NAVC); 2012. p. 873–9.

18. Hoenig M. Concurrent disease management: hyperthyroidism and diabetes mellitus. In: Little SE, editor. The cat: clinical medicine and management. St Louis (MO): Elsevier Saunders; 2012. p. 1101–3.

19. Peterson ME. Diagnosis and management of insulin resistance in dogs and cats with diabetes mellitus. Vet Clin North Am Small Anim Pract 1995;25:691–713. Available at: http://www.ncbi.nlm.nih.gov/pubmed/7660542.

20. Rand JS. Pathogenesis of feline diabetes. Vet Clin North Am Small Anim Pract 2013;43:221–31. Available at: http://www.ncbi.nlm.nih.gov/pubmed/23522168.

21. DiBartola SP, Rutgers HC, Zack PM, et al. Clinicopathologic findings associated with chronic renal disease in cats: 74 cases (1973-1984). J Am Vet Med Assoc 1987;190:1196–202. Available at: http://www.ncbi.nlm.nih.gov/pubmed/3583899.

22. Krawiec DR, Gelberg HB. Chronic renal disease in cats. In: Kirk RW, editor. Current veterinary therapy X. Philadelphia: W. B. Saunders Company; 1989. p. 1170–3.

23. Lulich JP, Osborne CA, O'Brien TD, et al. Feline renal failure: questions, answers, questions. Compend Cont Educ Pract Vet 1992;14:127–52.

24. Langston CE, Reine NJ. Hyperthyroidism and the kidney. Clin Tech Small Anim Pract 2006;21:17–21. Available at: http://www.ncbi.nlm.nih.gov/pubmed/16584026.

25. Syme HM. Cardiovascular and renal manifestations of hyperthyroidism. Vet Clin North Am Small Anim Pract 2007;37:723–43, vi. Available at: http://www.ncbi.nlm.nih.gov/pubmed/17619008.

26. Syme H. A common duo: hyperthyroidism and chronic kidney disease. Small Animal & Exotics Proceedings, Vol. 27. Gainesville (FL): North American Veterinary Conference (NAVC); 2013.

27. Williams TL. Is hyperthyroidism damaging to the feline kidney? [PhD thesis] London: Department of Veterinary Clinical Sciences: Royal Veterinary College, University of London; 2013.

28. Williams TL, Elliott J, Syme HM. Renin-angiotensin-aldosterone system activity in hyperthyroid cats with and without concurrent hypertension. J Vet Intern Med 2013;27:522–9. Available at: http://www.ncbi.nlm.nih.gov/pubmed/23517505.

29. Archer FJ, Taylor SM. Alkaline phosphatase bone isoenzyme and osteocalcin in the serum of hyperthyroid cats. Can Vet J 1996;37:735–9. Available at: http://www.ncbi.nlm.nih.gov/pubmed/9111692.

30. Barber PJ, Elliott J. Study of calcium homeostasis in feline hyperthyroidism. J Small Anim Pract 1996;37:575–82. Available at: http://www.ncbi.nlm.nih.gov/pubmed/8981278.

31. Schenck PA. Calcium homeostasis in thyroid disease in dogs and cats. Vet Clin North Am Small Anim Pract 2007;37:693–708, vi. Available at: http://www.ncbi.nlm.nih.gov/pubmed/17619006.

32. Williams TL, Elliott J, Syme HM. Calcium and phosphate homeostasis in hyperthyroid cats - associations with development of azotaemia and survival time. J Small Anim Pract 2012;53:561–71. Available at: http://www.ncbi.nlm.nih.gov/pubmed/22860883.

33. Barber PJ, Rawlings JM, Markwell PJ, et al. Effect of dietary phosphate restriction on renal secondary hyperparathyroidism in the cat. J Small Anim Pract 1999;40:62–70. Available at: http://www.ncbi.nlm.nih.gov/pubmed/10088085.

34. Elliott J, Rawlings JM, Markwell PJ, et al. Survival of cats with naturally occurring chronic renal failure: effect of dietary management. J Small Anim Pract 2000;41:235–42. Available at: http://www.ncbi.nlm.nih.gov/pubmed/10879400.

35. Fujita S, Volpi E. Nutrition and sarcopenia of ageing. Nutr Res Rev 2004;17:69–76. Available at: http://www.ncbi.nlm.nih.gov/pubmed/19079916.

36. Wolfe RR. Sarcopenia of aging: implications of the age-related loss of lean body mass. Proceedings of the Nestlé Purina Companion Animal Nutrition Summit: Focus on Gerontology. St. Louis (MO): Nestle Purina; 2010. p. 12–7. Available at: http://breedingbetterdogs.com/pdfFiles/articles/CAN2010_updated.pdf.

37. Sakuma K, Yamaguchi A. Sarcopenia and cachexia: the adaptations of negative regulators of skeletal muscle mass. J Cachexia Sarcopenia Muscle 2012;3:77–94. Available at: http://www.ncbi.nlm.nih.gov/pubmed/22476916.

38. Paddon-Jones D, Short KR, Campbell WW, et al. Role of dietary protein in the sarcopenia of aging. Am J Clin Nutr 2008;87:1562S–6S. Available at: http://www.ncbi.nlm.nih.gov/pubmed/18469288.

39. Little SE. Evaluation of the senior cat with weight loss. In: Little SE, editor. The cat: clinical medicine and management. St Louis (MO): Elsevier Saunders; 2012. p. 1176–81.

40. Patil AR, Cupp C, Pérez-Camargo G. Incidence of impaired nutrient digestibility in aging cats Nestlé Purina Nutrition Forum Proceedings. St. Louis (MO): Nestle Purina; 2003. p. 72.

41. Perez-Camargo G. Cat nutrition: what is new in the old? Compend Cont Educ Pract Vet 2004;26(Suppl 2A):5–10.

42. Wakshlag JJ. Dietary protein consumption in the healthy aging companion animal. Proceedings of the Nestlé Purina Companion Animal Nutrition Summit: Focus on Gerontology. St. Louis (MO): Nestle Purina; 2010. p. 32–9. Available at: http://breedingbetterdogs.com/pdfFiles/articles/CAN2010_updated.pdf.

43. Laflamme DP, Hannah SS. Discrepancy between use of lean body mass or nitrogen balance to determine protein requirements for adult cats. J Feline Med Surg 2013;15:691–7. Available at: http://www.ncbi.nlm.nih.gov/pubmed/23362342.

44. Laflamme D. Protein requirements of aging cats based on preservation of lean body mass. 13th Annual American Academy of Veterinary Nutrition (AAVN) Clinical Nutrition & Research Symposium. Seattle, Washington; June 12, 2013. p. 17.

45. Sparkes AH. Feeding old cats–an update on new nutritional therapies. Top Companion Anim Med 2011;26:37–42. Available at: http://www.ncbi.nlm.nih.gov/pubmed/21435625.

46. Vogt AH, Rodan I, Brown M, et al. AAFP-AAHA: feline life stage guidelines. J Am Anim Hosp Assoc 2010;46:70–85. Available at: http://www.ncbi.nlm.nih.gov/pubmed/20045841.

47. MacDonald ML, Rogers QR, Morris JG. Nutrition of the domestic cat, a mammalian carnivore. Annu Rev Nutr 1984;4:521–62. Available at: http://www.ncbi.nlm.nih.gov/pubmed/6380542.

48. Zoran DL. The carnivore connection to nutrition in cats. J Am Vet Med Assoc 2002;221:1559–67. Available at: http://www.ncbi.nlm.nih.gov/pubmed/12479324.

49. Eisert R. Hypercarnivory and the brain: protein requirements of cats reconsidered. J Comp Physiol B 2011;181:1–17. Available at: http://www.ncbi.nlm.nih.gov/pubmed/21088842.

50. Baral RM, Little SE. Endocrine pancreatic disorders. In: Little SE, editor. The cat: clinical medicine and management. St Louis (MO): Elsevier Saunders; 2012. p. 547–71.

51. Rucinsky R, Cook A, Haley S, et al. AAHA diabetes management guidelines. J Am Anim Hosp Assoc 2010;46:215–24. Available at: http://www.ncbi.nlm.nih.gov/pubmed/20439947.

52. Farrow H, Rand JS, Morton JM, et al. Postprandial glycemia in cats fed a moderate carbohydrate meal persists for a median of 12 hours – female cats have higher peak glucose concentrations. J Feline Med Surg 2012;14:706–15. Available at: http://www.ncbi.nlm.nih.gov/pubmed/22653915.

53. Farrow HA, Rand JS, Morton JM, et al. Effect of dietary carbohydrate, fat, and protein on postprandial glycemia and energy intake in cats. J Vet Intern Med 2013;27:1121–35. Available at: http://www.ncbi.nlm.nih.gov/pubmed/23869495.

54. Zoran DL, Rand JS. The role of diet in the prevention and management of feline diabetes. Vet Clin North Am Small Anim Pract 2013;43:233–43. Available at: http://www.ncbi.nlm.nih.gov/pubmed/23522169.

55. Kidder AC, Chew D. Treatment options for hyperphosphatemia in feline CKD: what's out there? J Feline Med Surg 2009;11:913–24. Available at: http://www.ncbi.nlm.nih.gov/pubmed/19857854.

56. Ross SJ, Osborne CA, Kirk CA, et al. Clinical evaluation of dietary modification for treatment of spontaneous chronic kidney disease in cats. J Am Vet Med Assoc 2006;229:949–57. Available at: http://www.ncbi.nlm.nih.gov/pubmed/16978113.

57. Geddes RF, Finch NC, Syme HM, et al. The role of phosphorus in the pathophysiology of chronic kidney disease. J Vet Emerg Crit Care (San Antonio) 2013;23:122–33. Available at: http://www.ncbi.nlm.nih.gov/pubmed/23464730.

58. International Renal Interest Society (IRIS). Staging of CKD. 2009. Available at: http://www.iris-kidney.com/guidelines/en/staging_ckd.shtml. Accessed April 13, 2013.

59. AAFCO (Association of American Feed Control Officials). 2014 official publication. Champaign (IL): AAFCO. 2014.

60. Elliott J. Hyperphosphataemia and chronic kidney disease - outcomes of the 2006 round table in Louiseville, KY (USA). State of the art in renal disease in cats and dogs. Nice (France): Vetoquinol Academia; 2007. p. 12–7. Available at: http://www.vetoquinolusa.com/Studies/CKD/StateOfTheArtProceedings.pdf.

61. Elliott KF, Rand JS, Fleeman LM, et al. A diet lower in digestible carbohydrate results in lower postprandial glucose concentrations compared with a traditional canine diabetes diet and an adult maintenance diet in healthy dogs. Res Vet Sci 2011;93:288–95. Available at: http://www.ncbi.nlm.nih.gov/pubmed/21944832.

62. Allen FM, Stillman E, Fitz RT. Total dietary regulation in the treatment of diabetes. Monographs of The Rockefeller Institute for Medical Research, Monograph No 11. New York: Rockefeller Institute for Medical Research; 1919. Available at: https://archive.org/details/cu31924104225283.

63. Lasker SP, McLachlan CS, Wang L, et al. Discovery, treatment and management of diabetes. J Diabetology 2010;1:1–8. Available at: http://www.journalofdiabetology. org/Pages/Releases/PDFFiles/FirstIssue/RA-1-JOD-09-001.pdf.

64. Vernon MC, Mavropoulos J, Transue M, et al. Clinical experience of a carbohydrate-restricted diet: effect on diabetes mellitus. Metab Syndr Relat Disord 2003;1:233–7. Available at: http://www.ncbi.nlm.nih.gov/pubmed/18370667.

65. Accurso A, Bernstein RK, Dahlqvist A, et al. Dietary carbohydrate restriction in type 2 diabetes mellitus and metabolic syndrome: time for a critical appraisal. Nutr Metab (Lond) 2008;9:5. Available at: http://www.ncbi.nlm.nih.gov/pubmed/18397522.

66. Westman EC, Yancy WS Jr, Mavropoulos JC, et al. The effect of a low-carbohydrate, ketogenic diet versus a low-glycemic index diet on glycemic control in type 2 diabetes mellitus. Nutr Metab (Lond) 2008;36:5. Available at: http://www.ncbi.nlm.nih.gov/pubmed/19099589.

67. Mori Y, Ohta T, Yokoyama J, et al. Effects of low-carbohydrate/high-monounsaturated fatty acid liquid diets on diurnal glucose variability and insulin dose in type 2 diabetes patients on tube feeding who require insulin therapy. Diabetes Technol Ther 2013;15:762–7. Available at: http://www.ncbi.nlm.nih.gov/pubmed/23931715.

68. Ajala O, English P, Pinkney J. Systematic review and meta-analysis of different dietary approaches to the management of type 2 diabetes. Am J Clin Nutr 2013;97:505–16. Available at: http://www.ncbi.nlm.nih.gov/pubmed/23364002.

69. Westman EC, Vernon MC. Has carbohydrate-restriction been forgotten as a treatment for diabetes mellitus? A perspective on the ACCORD study design. Nutr Metab (Lond) 2008;10:5. Available at: http://www.ncbi.nlm.nih.gov/pubmed/18400080.

70. Rand JS. Feline diabetes mellitus. In: Mooney CT, Peterson ME, editors. BSAVA manual of canine and feline endocrinology. 4th edition. Quedgeley (United Kingdom): British Small Animal Veterinary Association; 2012. p. 133–47.

71. Khemtemourian L, Killian JA, Hoppener JW, et al. Recent insights in islet amyloid polypeptide-induced membrane disruption and its role in beta-cell death in type 2 diabetes mellitus. Exp Diabetes Res 2008;2008:421287. Available at: http://www.ncbi.nlm.nih.gov/pubmed/18483616.

72. Link KR, Allio I, Rand JS, et al. The effect of experimentally induced chronic hyperglycaemia on serum and pancreatic insulin, pancreatic islet IGF-I and plasma and urinary ketones in the domestic cat (*Felis felis*). Gen Comp Endocrinol 2013;188:269–81. Available at: http://www.ncbi.nlm.nih.gov/pubmed/23660449.

73. Zini E, Osto M, Franchini M, et al. Hyperglycaemia but not hyperlipidaemia causes beta cell dysfunction and beta cell loss in the domestic cat. Diabetologia 2009;52:336–46. Available at: http://www.ncbi.nlm.nih.gov/pubmed/19034421.

74. Crenshaw KL, Peterson ME. Pretreatment clinical and laboratory evaluation of cats with diabetes mellitus: 104 cases (1992-1994). J Am Vet Med Assoc 1996;209:943–9. Available at: http://www.ncbi.nlm.nih.gov/pubmed/8790546.

75. Kim TN, Park MS, Yang SJ, et al. Prevalence and determinant factors of sarcopenia in patients with type 2 diabetes: the Korean Sarcopenic Obesity Study (KSOS). Diabetes Care 2010;33:1497–9. Available at: http://www.ncbi.nlm.nih.gov/pubmed/20413515.

76. Stenholm S, Harris TB, Rantanen T, et al. Sarcopenic obesity: definition, cause and consequences. Curr Opin Clin Nutr Metab Care 2008;11:693–700. Available at: http://www.ncbi.nlm.nih.gov/pubmed/18827572.

77. Srikanthan P, Hevener AL, Karlamangla AS. Sarcopenia exacerbates obesity-associated insulin resistance and dysglycemia: findings from the National Health and Nutrition Examination Survey III. PLoS One 2010;5:e10805. Available at: http://www.ncbi.nlm.nih.gov/pubmed/22421977.

78. Moon SS. Low skeletal muscle mass is associated with insulin resistance, diabetes, and metabolic syndrome in the Korean population: The Korea National Health and Nutrition Examination Survey (KNHANES) 2009-2010. Endocr J 2014;61(1):61–70. Available at: http://www.ncbi.nlm.nih.gov/pubmed/24088600.

79. Frank G, Anderson W, Pazak H, et al. Use of a high-protein diet in the management of feline diabetes mellitus. Vet Ther 2001;2:238–46. Available at: http://www.ncbi.nlm.nih.gov/pubmed/19746667.

80. Mazzaferro EM, Greco DS, Turner AS, et al. Treatment of feline diabetes mellitus using an alpha-glucosidase inhibitor and a low-carbohydrate diet. J Feline Med Surg 2003;5:183–9. Available at: http://www.ncbi.nlm.nih.gov/pubmed/12765629.

81. Bennett N, Greco DS, Peterson ME, et al. Comparison of a low carbohydrate-low fiber diet and a moderate carbohydrate-high fiber diet in the management of feline diabetes mellitus. J Feline Med Surg 2006;8:73–84. Available at: http://www.ncbi.nlm.nih.gov/pubmed/16275041.

82. Boari A, Aste G, Rocconi F, et al. Glargine insulin and high-protein-low-carbohydrate diet in cats with diabetes mellitus. Vet Res Commun 2008;32(Suppl 1):S243–5. Available at: http://www.ncbi.nlm.nih.gov/pubmed/18685984.

83. Roomp K, Rand J. Intensive blood glucose control is safe and effective in diabetic cats using home monitoring and treatment with glargine. J Feline Med Surg 2009;11:668–82. Available at: http://www.ncbi.nlm.nih.gov/pubmed/19592286.

84. Roomp K, Rand J. Evaluation of detemir in diabetic cats managed with a protocol for intensive blood glucose control. J Feline Med Surg 2012;14:566–72. Available at: http://www.ncbi.nlm.nih.gov/pubmed/22553309.

85. Marshall RD, Rand JS, Morton JM. Treatment of newly diagnosed diabetic cats with glargine insulin improves glycaemic control and results in higher probability of remission than protamine zinc and lente insulins. J Feline Med Surg 2009;11:683–91. Available at: http://www.ncbi.nlm.nih.gov/pubmed/19539509.

86. Nguyen P, Leray V, Dumon H, et al. High protein intake affects lean body mass but not energy expenditure in nonobese neutered cats. J Nutr 2004;134:2084S–6S. Available at: http://www.ncbi.nlm.nih.gov/pubmed/15284408.

87. Keller U. Dietary proteins in obesity and in diabetes. Int J Vitam Nutr Res 2011;81:125–33. Available at: http://www.ncbi.nlm.nih.gov/pubmed/22139563.

Pet Obesity Management
Beyond Nutrition

Deborah Linder, DVM[a],*, Megan Mueller, PhD[b]

KEYWORDS

- Obesity • Nutrition • Weight management • Client communication
- Human-animal interaction • Human-animal bond

KEY POINTS

- Obesity is a complex and multifactorial condition that is easier to prevent than treat.
- Successful weight management plans for pets incorporate diet, exercise, and an understanding of human-animal interaction.
- Compliance increases when plans are tailored to meet the needs of each individual pet, owner, and environment.
- Understanding the complex and unique connection between owners and their pets allows successful weight management and long-term client trust.

 Video of successful weight management strategy in an 8-year-old dog accompanies this article at http://www.vetsmall.theclinics.com/

INTRODUCTION

Obesity is a multifactorial condition that needs to be treated as a complex nutritional disorder requiring comprehensive management. Despite initiating standard diet and exercise, many weight management plans in the authors' experience fail because of veterinarians and pet owners not acknowledging and addressing the complex nature of obesity. Successful weight management programs extend beyond standard nutritional management and incorporate an understanding of human-animal interaction. This understanding is developed with effective client communication that helps the veterinary team better appreciate each family's unique relationship with its pet and how diet and exercise can be incorporated into their environment. Thus, obesity

Disclosure: Dr D. Linder's faculty appointment is funded by a grant from Royal Canin, USA. Dr M. Mueller's faculty appointment is funded in part by Zoetis.

[a] Department of Clinical Sciences, Cummings School of Veterinary Medicine at Tufts University, 200 Westboro Road, North Grafton, MA 01536, USA; [b] Center for Animals and Public Policy, Cummings School of Veterinary Medicine at Tufts University, 200 Westboro Road, North Grafton, MA 01536, USA
* Corresponding author.
E-mail address: deborah.linder@tufts.edu

treatment requires management from both medical and social science perspectives to achieve success. Obesity is a condition requiring lifelong management; however, when veterinarians go beyond standard treatment to incorporate each pet owner's unique relationship with their pet into the plan, it is also in the authors' opinion one of the few diseases in veterinary medicine that can be completely preventable and curable.

The Status of Pet Obesity

Obesity is one of the most common health problems affecting dogs and cats, with an estimated 34% to 59% of dogs[1–3] and 25% to 63% of cats[4–8] being overweight or obese. The most common and clinically applicable method of diagnosing obesity is assessing a body condition score (BCS). A 9-point, 5-point, or lettering system can be used, as long as the same system is used consistently and explained to staff and pet owners. BCS is only used to assess body fat, whereas muscle condition scoring (MCS) is used to quantify muscle wasting.[9] MCS is a monitoring technique to help veterinarians monitor for muscle wasting during weight management. Each BCS on a 9-point scale is generally associated with a 10% to 15% increase or decrease from ideal body weight and can help determine ideal weight for that pet.[10–12] Although definitions of obesity vary, overweight is generally considered to be 10% to 20% more than optimal body weight (BCS of 6–7 out of 9) and obese as 20% or greater more than optimal body weight (BCS of 7–9 out of 9). Pets with a BCS 7 out of 9 could be considered either overweight or obese. Body weight, BCS, and MCS should be a standard part of every physical examination and should be documented at every veterinary visit.

Risk Factors for Obesity

Risk factors for pet obesity vary in studies conducted worldwide on dogs and cats (**Table 1**). One epidemiologic study found that the risk factors for obesity in dogs were almost exclusively owner related, such as owner age, frequency of treats, amount of exercise, and owner income, which was also associated with lower awareness of obesity-related health risks.[3] Many owner-related and husbandry risk factors for obesity highlight the need for veterinarians to fully understand the environment of the pet, as well as how the family dynamics and the pet-owner relationship may affect weight status and effectiveness of interventions.

Table 1
Risk factors associated with obesity

Cat	Dog
Neutering	Neutering
Cat breed	Dog breed
Cat age	Dog age
Male sex	Frequency and type of treats (table scraps)
Owner age	Owner age
Food type (premium, therapeutic, high fat)	Food type (noncommercial, canned)
Frequency of feeding	Frequency of feeding
Sedentary or inactive lifestyle/exercise	Sedentary or inactive lifestyle/exercise
Indoor housing	Owner income
Owner underestimation of cat's BCS	—

Data from Refs.[1–8,13–15,75]

Perception of Obesity

Also noted as a risk factor for obesity was the pet owner's underestimation of the pet's BCS. In 2 separate studies, 39% of owners underestimated their pet's BCS, even after knowing their veterinarian's assessment of BCS.[16,17] Further evidence of misperception among pet owners was shown in a study by Bland and colleagues,[18] in which half of the owners who correctly identified their pets' BCS score at more than ideal weight still did not consider their pet to be overweight. This discrepancy of views of body condition may stem from public perception of breed standards that an overweight condition is the standard of beauty; one study on show dogs revealed that almost 1 in every 5 show dogs was overweight.[19] Owner perception also factors into pet feeding practices and adherence to weight management plans. Studies have shown that the size of the food bowl and food scoop affects the amount of food owners feed their dogs,[20] and even veterinary staff's accuracy of feeding a specific amount of food varied from an 18% underestimate to an 80% overestimate of the intended amount.[21] With many owner-related risk factors for obesity combined with a misperception of body condition and feeding practices, weight management in pets requires comprehensive treatment that includes the owner and extends beyond the standard diet and exercise regimen.

CLINICAL CONSIDERATIONS IN OBESITY
Client Cost for Obesity

Although studies in veterinary medicine are lacking, one study projects that, by 2030, costs could range from US$860.7 billion to US$956.9 billion spent on health care attributable to overweight or obesity in humans.[22] Owners with financial concerns should be made aware of the possible increased costs associated with having an overweight pet, which can include food, veterinary care, medications, and associated comorbidities. Irrespective of finances, obese patients require special clinical consideration.

Adjusted Body Weight and Medication Dosage

Drug dosages are of particular importance in medications with a narrow safety range, such as some chemotherapeutics and immunosuppressive medications. Calculating requirements based on obese body weight may increase risk of side effects, whereas using ideal weight is more subjective and could potentially lead to decreased efficacy. Each patient and medication must be considered on an individual basis. Obese patients undergoing anesthesia may be at higher risk and should be monitored and dosed carefully. Although studies in human medicine have started assessing the problem of dosages for obese patients,[23] more studies are needed in veterinary medicine to determine the most efficacious way to adjust body weight and dose medications. Discussing these additional risks incurred because of excess weight at the time of anesthesia or medication dosing can remind owners of the current consequences of obesity in their pets, especially if they are not yet encountering clinical signs from their pets' obesity.

CONSEQUENCES OF OBESITY

Although pet owners may not be worried about the social stigma of obesity, being overweight has been associated with many clinical and subclinical conditions that put a pet's health at risk. Without prospective randomized clinical trials, much of the epidemiologic information in veterinary medicine can only provide an association between obesity and diseases, not a direct causation. However, as more evidence accumulates on the associations between excess weight and diseases, there is an indication that being lean is likely healthier.

Subclinical Consequences of Obesity

Although it was once thought that adipose tissue was metabolically inert, evidence increasingly suggests that adipose tissue produces hormones and inflammatory mediators (eg, adipokines such as leptin) that can have considerable clinical and subclinical effects on the body.[24,25] These effects can manifest as predisposing pets to diseases or exacerbating current diseases through a proinflammatory process (ie, adipose tissue producing inflammatory cytokines such as tumor necrosis factor alpha and interleukin-6).[25] Obesity can predispose pets to endocrine diseases, and in dogs it has been related to hypercholesterolemia, hypertriglyceridemia, hyperinsulinemia, increased leptin, and decreased ghrelin.[26] In cats, obesity is associated with impaired insulin sensitivity, even in cats younger than 1 year of age,[27] highlighting the need for preventative and aggressive weight management before pets are obese with clinical disease. Subclinical conditions are challenging to discuss with pet owners because the consequences are not readily apparent; however, before clinical signs are evident is the ideal time to address weight management.

Clinical Diseases Associated with Obesity

Obesity has been associated with numerous diseases, most notably diabetes and osteoarthritis, in which excess weight not only predisposes to this condition but in which weight loss can improve these conditions.[28,29] Approaching weight management not as an option or adjunct treatment but as a standard of care and treatment in these diseases helps pet owners and the veterinary staff to reach the critical goals of maintaining and achieving a healthy weight, as well as reducing disease symptoms. Many other diseases, involving almost every body system, have also been associated with excess weight in companion animals (**Table 2**). Pet owners are familiar with many of these associations in human medicine and discussing these risks as analogous to human health concerns can help with owner comprehension and acceptance of the severity of obesity in their animals. In addition, even moderate amounts of excess weight may contribute to a shorter lifespan. In a lifetime study, a group of Labrador retrievers maintained at a median BCS of 4 to 5 out of 9 lived a median of 1.8 years longer than a control group maintained at a median BCS of 6 to 7 out of 9.[32] Obesity in all species is more easily prevented than treated and the entire veterinary team plays an important role in educating and guiding clients before the pet becomes obese.

Quality of Life in Obese Pets

Anecdotal evidence and studies show that pet owners have expressed guilt or fear of depriving their pet of food as a rationale for not engaging in weight loss plans. However, data now support that pets have a decreased quality of life when overweight and improve in these measures (such as vitality, emotional disturbance, and pain) after successful weight loss.[33] Discussing the quality-of-life consequences of obesity and the benefits of weight loss may help alleviate owner hesitancy in initiating and implementing weight management plans. In addition, although pet owners may find it challenging to associate current obesity with clinical disease repercussions in the future, veterinarians can emphasize effects on a pet's current quality of life that may be adversely affected by obesity.

PREVENTION

An important part of initial puppy and kitten visits includes a discussion of proper feeding and BCS with pet owners.[64,65] Owners should be instructed to quantify and measure the food they feed their pets to achieve an ideal body condition, rather

Table 2
Conditions reported to be associated with obesity in cats and dogs

Body System	Condition	Species
Overall	Anesthetic/surgical risk	Dog
	Reduced longevity	Dog
	Reduced quality of life	Dog
Immune	Decreased immune function, susceptibility to infection	Dog
Endocrine	Impaired glucose tolerance	Cat
	Diabetes	Dog, cat
	Insulin resistance, hyperinsulinemia	Dog
	Dyslipidemia, hypercholesterolemia, hypertriglyceridemia	Dog, cat
	Pancreatitis	Dog
	Hypothyroidism	Dog
Orthopedic	Degenerative joint disease, hip dysplasia	Dog
	Osteoarthritis, chronic lameness	Dog, cat
	Humeral condylar fractures, cranial cruciate rupture	Dog
	Intervertebral disc disease	Dog
Cardiorespiratory	Cardiac alterations	Cat, dog
	Heart rate and function	Dog
	Tracheal collapse	Dog
	Airway dysfunction	Dog
	Heatstroke	Dog
Neoplasia	Neoplasia	Dog, cat
	Mammary neoplasia	Dog
	Urinary neoplasia	Dog
Urogenital	Renal alterations	Dog
	Lower urinary tract disease, urolithiasis	Dog, cat
Integument	Dermatitis	Cat
Dental	Oral disease	Dog, cat

Data from Refs.[2,5,26,30–63]

than free feeding. This distinction is particularly important for large-breed puppies, for which a BCS of 4 to 5 on a 9-point scale has been shown to be ideal.[32] A puppy or kitten food lower in caloric density should be selected, if needed, rather than switching to an adult food to ensure that all essential nutrients are provided during growth. In many pets, energy requirements decrease after spaying or neutering,[66] and a discussion with pet owners is needed at the time of spay or neuter to monitor their pets' BCS and reduce intake if necessary. Weight management and obesity prevention are lifelong; prevention is best achieved in the authors' experience with discussions on BCS and consistent monitoring for risk factors at yearly wellness visits with nutritional assessments. Methods for performing a full nutritional assessment are described elsewhere.[64,65] Feeding directions, even on foods marketed for weight management, can grossly overestimate the energy requirements of a cat or dog,[67] so owners should continue to feed to an ideal body condition at all life stages.

INITIAL APPROACH TO WEIGHT MANAGEMENT
Pet Assessment

A physical examination, nutritional assessment, and diagnostic work-up as appropriate can determine any health conditions that may affect development or implementation of a weight loss plan (eg, comorbid disease, exercise intolerance). BCS and

MCS should be a crucial part of every patient examination. When evaluating dogs and cats on these scores, veterinarians may note that not all pets have similar BCS and MCS (eg, an obese pet, which would be a BCS 9 on a 9-point scale, could also have severe muscle wasting). After a patient examination, a complete and thorough diet history allows an accurate estimate of daily caloric intake, and examples of diet history forms have been published previously.[64,65] Many owners are not aware that supplements, treats, rawhides, or dental chews contain calories, so these should specifically be discussed.

Owner Assessment

After assessing the pet and obtaining a complete diet history, taking time to understand the environment and pet owners allows assessment of the owner's readiness to change and ability to commit to a weight loss program. Some pet owners may not be ready and are still contemplating weight management, in which case client education and monitoring are best received. However, those preparing or taking action for weight management may best benefit from specific individualized plans and feedback. Talking tips and further information about assessing readiness to change has been described elsewhere.[68] Some examples of talking points are included in **Box 1**. By understanding clients' background, weight management can be approached by the veterinarian in a way clients will accept and engage in for optimal success.

SELECTING A DIET: NUTRIENTS OF CONCERN

Recommending that pet owners select for themselves over-the-counter diets marketed for weight management is not ideal, because these diets vary considerably in calorie density (eg, ranging from 217–480 kcal/cup for dry cat and dog food) and feeding directions.[67] If feeding an over-the-counter food is warranted or the only option for the pet owner, then it can be helpful to guide the owner by making a specific product recommendation or providing specific criteria to meet each patient's needs (eg, guidelines for calorie density, protein concentration in diet, and so forth). The optimal nutrient profile for a weight loss diet is based on medical factors as well as the preferences and lifestyle of the owner and the pet. Compliance is critical in weight management, and paying particular attention to owners' concerns in diet selection increases success.

Box 1
Talking points for veterinarians when discussing weight management with clients

- What are your thoughts on your pet's weight?
- It sounds like you are concerned that your pet's weight may be limiting your pet's ability to play with your other pets.
- How do the other members in your household feel about a possible weight loss plan for your pet?
- You are right to be concerned about your pet's weight and you did the right thing bringing your pet in today to discuss it.
- Weight loss can be challenging and we may need to adjust our plan, but we are here to help you through it.
- How could we work together to overcome the challenge of feeding multiple pets?
- What challenges do you anticipate in implementing our weight management plan for your pet?

Lower Calorie Density

Methods for reducing calorie density include reduced fat, added moisture, or added fiber. One study showed short-term decreased voluntary intake and body weight in cats fed ad libitum with increased dietary water content.[69] This benefit of added moisture may differ for each pet and may be prohibitively expensive for some owners, depending on the method (ie, adding water vs purchasing canned food). Studies on fiber and satiety have been conflicting, with some reporting increased satiety,[70,71] whereas others have shown no benefit.[72,73] Although many cats and dogs do well on high-fiber diets, some may have gastrointestinal side effects such as vomiting or diarrhea, and gradual introduction is recommend to minimize these side effects. Discussing possible side effects and potential for increased fecal volume and frequency with pet owners helps avoid compliance concerns during weight loss.

Macronutrient Profile (Protein, Carbohydrates, and Fat)

Many therapeutic weight management foods have a low fat content, although this is not required. Increased protein may have a role in satiety,[71] but, more importantly, it has been shown to help retain lean body mass during weight loss.[74] The goal of providing increased protein is to reduce the need for animals to break down their own muscle to meet essential protein needs, but protein can also promote fat loss and aids in reducing weight rebound. There is no evidence to support that high-carbohydrate diets lead to obesity in cats. On the contrary, high-fat diets have been shown experimentally to be more of a concern for obesity development than high-carbohydrate diets when free fed.[75]

Micronutrient Profile

Weight loss diets should be selected that contain an increased nutrient/calorie ratio and have been formulated for weight loss. Restricting the amount of over-the-counter maintenance food that is fed, especially diets with high caloric densities, may not provide satiety for most pets because of volume restriction, which can contribute to poor adherence to the plan. In addition, restricting amounts of over-the-counter maintenance diets, including some marketed for weight management, could also lead to deficiency of one or more essential nutrients.[76] Further studies are needed to determine optimal nutrient requirements for overweight animals, although preliminary studies suggest minimal risk when using purpose-formulated therapeutic weight loss diets.[77]

Additional Nutrients

Some weight loss diets have additional components such as carnitine, a cofactor in fat metabolism; omega-3 fatty acids; soy isoflavonoids; or medium chain triglycerides. At this time, there is little to no evidence to show that any nutritional supplement aids in weight loss[78]; further research is needed before widespread supplementation can be recommended.

Treats

Providing treats is a central component of many pet owners' relationships with their pets, particularly in dogs. In one study, owners considered veterinary guidance, diet modification, a veterinary weight loss product, increase of exercise, and attending an obesity clinic before they considered eliminating treats to get their pet to lose weight.[79] Understanding this human-animal interaction (discussed later) allows a more realistic weight loss plan to be devised that can preserve the pet-owner relationship without compromising weight loss. Weight management plans can include treats, but they should be discussed and limited to not more than 10% of the total calorie intake. Some examples of low-calorie treats include nonstarch vegetables such as carrots or celery. As an alternative, small portions of the daily allotment of food can be given throughout the day as treats.

ENERGY RESTRICTION
Initial Calculation

Starting points for caloric restriction vary.[32,80–82] If current intake can be obtained or estimated from a complete diet history, then a 20% restriction from that can be a starting amount.[81] However, in the case of ad libitum feeding or when current intake cannot be estimated, the starting point varies from resting energy requirement (RER; 70 kcal/$kg^{0.75}$) for current weight to RER for ideal weight to a percentage of the maintenance energy requirement for current or ideal weight.[81] Using RER for current weight may not provide adequate caloric restriction to ensure weight loss,[82] and estimating ideal weight is complicated by subjectivity, especially in extremely obese animals. However, the calculated RER for an estimated target weight can be a starting point from which the necessary adjustments can be made. More important than the starting caloric amount are biweekly or monthly weigh-ins to ensure a safe and effective rate of weight loss. Preparing owners for the likely adjustments at each weigh-in helps manage client expectations during the program.

Rate of Weight Loss

The aim of initial energy allocation is to ensure that the rate of weight loss is steady, but the target rate of weight loss is likely to depend on the pet and situation. In studies, rates of weight loss range from 0.5% to 2% of weekly body weight loss for cats and dogs,[72,80] with a median rate of 0.85% per week (range of 0.35%–1.56%) in one study of client-owned dogs.[83] In addition, one study showed that 1% of body weight loss per week limited risk of nutrient deficiency, loss of lean body mass, and rebound weight gain.[74] Adjusting rate of weight loss and caloric restriction requires frequent follow-up and owners should be prepared for multiple weigh-ins to adequately align expectations and time frame for weight loss. For some cat owners, purchasing a baby scale to avoid frequent stressful trips to the veterinary clinic may prove useful. It is common for pets to plateau eventually in their weight loss as well, and this aspect should be included in early discussions on owner expectations for weight management (see **Box 1**). Additional strategies for common weight management challenges can be found in the 2014 AAHA Weight Management Guidelines (https://www.aahanet.org/library/WeightManagement.aspx).

Special Considerations

Exceptions to the range of weight loss rates discussed earlier include dogs and cats with comorbidities in which a more gradual rate of loss (0.5%) is recommended, although further studies are needed to determine target rates in various disease conditions. In addition, cats and dogs often decrease their energy requirements significantly when faced with caloric restriction.[80,84] In these situations in which cats and dogs require severe caloric restriction for weight loss, it may be even more important to ensure appropriate diet selection to provide adequate essential nutrients and to prepare owners for the necessity of further restrictions.

Energy Restriction for Maintenance of Weight Loss

Once ideal weight has been reached, most cats and dogs need ongoing calorie control and careful monitoring of body condition. Because of many pets' low energy requirements to maintain target body condition even after weight loss, diets with high nutrient/calorie ratios should be considered for these cats and dogs. Reinduction of obesity occurs more easily and faster with pets that have previously been over-weight,[85] so lifelong monitoring of caloric intake is required in most cases and owners should be counseled and prepared for transition to this maintenance phase.

PHYSICAL ACTIVITY FOR MANAGEMENT OF OBESITY

After patient assessment to determine suitability for physical activity, exercise can be an integral part of a weight loss program. Increased physical activity has been shown to allow dogs to ingest slightly more calories while maintaining weight loss goals.[86] With the exception of walking, information on other forms of exercise in pets is largely undocumented. Any increase in physical activity is likely to be beneficial for pets; how-ever, the benefits are difficult to quantify because of a lack of research. Owners should be encouraged to increase their pets' activity gradually, starting with 5 to 10 minutes per day with creative and low-intensity activities (such as walking or swimming) for previously sedentary pets. For pets with exercise limitations (such as dogs with ortho-pedic disease), there are an increasing number of veterinary physical rehabilitation services available that can help improve strength and mobility while limiting the risk of further injury. More studies are showing potential benefit from physical therapy and aquatic therapy as a part of a weight management program as well.[87,88] Encour-aging exercise in cats can include spreading meals throughout different parts of the house or use of food-dispensing toys, interactive toys, laser pointers, and electronic mice. Further ideas for feline-specific activities are described elsewhere.[89] An impor-tant aspect of creating a physical activity program and recommendations is dis-cussing and deciding with the pet owner any limitations of the pet or owner, expectations, schedule, and potential challenges (such as the winter months in colder climates or dog walker availability).

HOW TO INTEGRATE HUMAN-ANIMAL INTERACTION INTO OBESITY PREVENTION AND TREATMENT

An important facet of successful weight management is the role that human-animal relationships can play in affecting obesity prevention and treatment. Owners may need social and psychological support in addition to veterinary medical support in implementing weight management plans. Understanding the processes and dynamics of human-animal relationships can be useful for practitioners in developing successful treatment plans for their clients. The process of putting social science theory into prac-tice is discussed later with scenarios and practical management examples of the psy-chosocial aspects of a weight management program being incorporated into standard nutritional management.

The Discussion of Pet Obesity

Veterinarians who are uncomfortable having a conversation about obesity are not alone, because many health care providers for humans are hesitant to communicate about weight management with their patients.[90] Human obesity and its related health conditions represent a serious and growing public health concern that parallels pet obesity, with a tripling of human obesity incidence in the past 30 years.[91] Similar to veterinary medicine, the development of effective and sustainable interventions to treat obesity and prevent health sequelae such as heart disease and diabetes remains both a priority and a challenge in human medicine. Also similar to addressing human weight loss, the health care provider's approach to each pet owner may need to be different. It can be helpful to base this approach on the owners' interactions and relationships with their pets as a part of prioritizing a conversation about weight management. Three scenarios are included here with additional examples in **Box 1**.

- Educational example: in the authors' experience, some pet owners have been upset that previous veterinarians had not mentioned that their pets' weight was a potential health risk and assumed their pets were a normal or healthy weight based on their veterinarians' lack of concern. To avoid this, asking whether anyone has ever discussed the pet's weight with them before or whether anyone has discussed with them the risk of diabetes in overweight cats can be a casual start to a conversation that normalizes the problem and addresses health information in a neutral way.
- Comparison example: owners who are overweight often bring up their weight or similar struggles they are experiencing with obesity once the topic is introduced. Although it is not recommended for veterinarians to provide weight management advice for humans, drawing on similarities may prove helpful. For example, if an owner were to say, "I know I'd rather have a cookie than kibble," a potential response could be, "In moderation, treats are fine, but, just like us, our pets could get sick if they ate only candy or cookies all the time. Would you like to discuss a possible weight management plan that includes balanced food and treats that your pet likes?"
- Emotional example: some pet owners have a strong emotional attachment to their pets, with 70% of pet owners saying that their animals are sometimes allowed to sleep in their beds, and many note that they buy their pets presents, cook meals for them, and dress them up.[92] Resistance to discussing weight management can be heard in some client statements such as, "It would be cruel to 'starve' my pet and not give him whatever food he wants." These emotional statements can be addressed by an explanation of the impact of weight loss, explaining that weight loss is not emotionally hurtful to pets and does not cause them pain. The opposite is true: overweight pets are more likely to be in pain and can have emotional disturbance.[33] Weight loss makes them feel better.

Creating Effective Weight Management Plans by Understanding Owner-Pet Attachment

Pet ownership, and attachment in particular, have been linked to a host of beneficial human mental health outcomes.[93] The benefits of interacting with animals can include increased empathy,[94] a sense of emotional support,[95] and reduction of loneliness[96] and stress.[97] Given that owners can have such depth in their relationships with their pets such that their mental health is positively affected, weight management programs that affect this connection must be tailored to preserve that beneficial relationship. Understanding pet owners' attachment to their pets helps to build trust between the health care team and the pet owner. Building on this trust, weight management plans can be created with pet owners that strengthen their relationship with their pets and do not threaten their bonds.

Strong feelings of attachment may affect what owners are willing to do, influencing treatment in both positive and negative ways. For example, owners who are highly attached to their pets may be more willing to devote financial resources and time to obtaining veterinary care and adhering to a weight management plan. However, high levels of attachment may also be associated with emotional dependency. An owner who has a strong emotional relationship with an animal may be less inclined to withhold food or treats that may represent a part of that relationship. For example, when creating a weight management plan, veterinarians could ask, "Would you describe your daily routine that you and your pet share?" or "Is there anything you feel strongly about including in our plan?" In the authors' experience, these questions can often reveal nonnegotiables that can be incorporated to make owners feel more comfortable with the plan. For example, if an owner says that every night before bed the pet needs to have a chew treat while the owner reads in bed, a compromise can be made in terms of the type of treat in order to preserve that aspect of their relationship while adhering to a weight management plan. In another scenario, an owner acknowledges that it may be emotionally challenging to initiate exercise with a pet that does not seem to enjoy physical activity. **Box 2** and Video 1 explain how an understanding of the emotional attachment between the owner and pet can help the client devise ways to address these challenges and still be successful in weight loss.

Box 2
Successful weight management strategy: case example Mimi

History: Mimi, an 8-year-old spayed female mixed-breed dog, presented for a weight management consultation after a recent diagnosis of osteoarthritis and intermittent episodes of back pain. Other than mild to moderate pain on limb extension, a physical examination and screening laboratory work did not reveal significant abnormalities. Mimi was 15.9 kg (35 lb) with a BCS of 7/9, normal muscle condition, and an estimated 12.2 kg (27 lb) ideal weight. A diet history revealed that Mimi was being fed 500 kcal/d of an adult maintenance canine dry food as well as approximately 150 kcal/d in treats including multiple biscuits and a rawhide. Cheese and deli meat were used to administer an antiinflammatory medication twice daily, which added an additional 100 kcal/d.

Initial plan: because a complete diet history was obtained and a total caloric intake of 750 kcal was estimated, a 20% reduction in total caloric intake (600 kcal) was initiated with a therapeutic weight loss food (540 kcal) with 10% reserved for treats (60 kcal). Mimi was initially placed on exercise restriction for 4 weeks and monitored for any further episodes of back pain. During this time, her weight management plan consisted solely of dietary management and she was weighed weekly and her food intake was adjusted to meet a goal rate of weight loss (0.5%–1% of weight loss per week).

Incorporating human-animal interaction into management: 1 month later, Mimi had lost 450 g (1 lb) and was able to start a gradually increasing physical activity program. Discussing the plan with the owner, there was significant concern that Mimi did not enjoy physical activity and only got excited at meal time. Even though she was receiving a larger volume of food on the therapeutic diet, she ate her food quickly and enthusiastically, but then went back to being sedentary until the next meal. On further discussion, the owner also felt guilty over forcing Mimi to exercise with walks or water therapy when he thought that she did not like it and he did not want his dog to resent him or their time together.

Preserving the relationship: seeing Mimi show enthusiasm and enjoy their time together was an important aspect of the relationship between the owner and Mimi. For both the owner and Mimi to benefit from positive interaction, Mimi's food motivation was encouraged as a time to explore creative ways to interact incorporating physical activity. Instead of allowing Mimi to eat all her food quickly, the owner started placing the food in different areas of the house and allowed Mimi to search for and find her food. The owner was able to see Mimi enjoy walking from room to room and excitedly finding parts of her meal.

Follow-up: Mimi is currently a 5/9 BCS with an ideal weight of 11.3 kg (25 lb). Both the owner and Mimi look forward to meal time as a way to positively interact and improve the mental and physical health of both the pet and the owner. The owner is no longer anxious or worried about Mimi not enjoying physical activity and also has been creative in being more active himself at her mealtime.

Incorporating Family Dynamics to Address Challenges in Weight Management Plans

Understanding the nature of the human-animal relationships in a particular family setting can help the veterinarian develop an appropriate weight management program that is feasible to implement within the existing family dynamics. When collecting a diet history and discussing the potential plan, owners should also be asked about their relationships with their pets and how this relates to the other members of the family and their relationships with the pet. It can be useful to ask clients specific questions about which family member(s) are responsible for various aspects of the pet's care (eg, feeding, exercise, veterinary care, grooming). This information may help the veterinarian develop a weight management plan that fits into the existing family structure, and capitalizes on the owner-pet relationship that already exists. In addition, knowledge of the family human-animal relationships helps identify and preemptively address any potential barriers to weight management plan adherence. **Box 3** presents a scenario in which an accurate diet history was obtained only after including the entire family. Addressing the needs of all the family members with respect to their relationships with the pet led to successful weight loss.

Box 3
Successful weight management strategy: case example Kane

History: Kane presented as an overweight 5-year-old neutered male Labrador retriever for a weight management plan. Kane was 44 kg (97 lb) on presentation with a BCS of 8/9 and normal muscle condition. A full physical examination and wellness laboratory work revealed no significant abnormalities and his ideal weight was estimated to be 31.8 kg (70 lb). An initial diet history revealed that he was receiving 600 kcal/d from an over-the-counter weight management dry dog food and additional unknown calories from table scraps with each meal, which varied daily depending on what the family had for dinner.

Initial plan: at first, the family was switched to a therapeutic weight loss food given Kane's need for caloric restriction, and the total caloric amount was reduced by 20%. On a first recheck 2 weeks later, Kane had not lost any weight.

Incorporating human-animal interaction into management: when weight loss was not successful, the patient was referred to a specialist for weight management assessment. With a complete diet history, the human-animal interaction of the family environment was also assessed. On further discussion, it was discovered that there were 3 teenage girls in the household, along with 2 parents, all of whom had differing daily schedules and who thought it was their responsibility to feed Kane and provide additional treats. Throughout the day, Kane was fed at least one additional meal not disclosed on the initial diet history and he was receiving approximately 400 kcal in various biscuits, chews, and table scraps throughout the day.

Preserving the relationship: when all family members were present, a daily feeding schedule was discussed for Kane that included 1000 kcal total with 900 kcal in a therapeutic weight loss food (RER for ideal weight) and 10% of the total 1000 kcal (100 kcal) reserved for Kane's favorite treats. In order to ensure that Kane was not fed multiple times or fed more than this amount, a food box allowance was prepared nightly for the following day that included a variety of treats and his meals adding up to 1000 kcal. Everyone in the family was able to see that Kane received a lot of treats and food throughout the day; it was simply spread out among many family members.

Follow-up: Kane is currently at 35 kg (77 lb) on monthly rechecks and the family is continuing to follow the agreed-on plan. All family members, including the children in the house, still feel connected to Kane and are able to maintain a special relationship by providing treats without compromising on his essential weight management.

PARTNERING WITH PETS TO ACHIEVE WELLNESS

One study[98] has shown that a weight loss program in pets can have a positive impact on their owners who may also be trying to lose weight. In addition, overweight pet owners may have a stronger attachment to their pets and have less perceived social support from humans than healthy-weight pet owners.[99] All pet owners can increase their bonds with their pets through healthy exercise instead of through extra calories in treats, which is how some owners express their love. Future research into integrative treatment programs is warranted to target human and animal health, such as family-oriented obesity treatment programs in which overweight families and their pets can become healthy together. These types of programs have immense potential for significantly affecting health and wellness in veterinary and human medicine through a focus on preserving beneficial healthy human-animal relationships.

SUMMARY

Many risk factors, combined with complexity in human-animal interaction, can create an environment conducive to pet obesity. Likewise, integrating the medical and social science aspects of obesity can lead to successful weight management. Although obesity requires intensive and comprehensive management, there are many novel aspects of obesity treatment, even many yet to be investigated, that can lead to a rewarding and enriching owner and veterinarian experience. Early intervention prevents challenging obesity treatment and provides pets with the best quality of life. Weight management requires a comprehensive approach that includes understanding and addressing the complex relationship of owners with their pets beyond the standard nutritional management for success.

SUPPLEMENTARY DATA

Supplementary data related to this article can be found online at http://dx.doi.org/10.1016/j.cvsm.2014.03.004.

REFERENCES

1. McGreevy PD, Thomson PC, Pride C, et al. Prevalence of obesity in dogs examined by Australian veterinary practices and the risk factors involved. Vet Rec 2005;156(22):695–702.
2. Lund EM, Armstrong PJ, Kirk CA, et al. Prevalence and risk factors for obesity in adult dogs from private US veterinary practices. Intern J Appl Res Vet Med 2006;4(2):177–86.
3. Courcier EA, Thomson RM, Mellor DJ, et al. An epidemiological study of environmental factors associated with canine obesity. J Small Anim Pract 2010;51(7):362–7.
4. Scarlett JM, Donoghue S, Saidla J, et al. Overweight cats: prevalence and risk factors. Int J Obes 1994;18(S1):S22–8.
5. Lund EM, Armstrong PJ, Kirk CA, et al. Prevalence and risk factors for obesity in adult cats from private US veterinary practices. Intern J Appl Res Vet Med 2005;3(2):88–96.
6. Colliard L, Paragon BM, Lemuet B, et al. Prevalence and risk factors of obesity in an urban population of healthy cats. J Feline Med Surg 2009;11(2):135–40.
7. Courcier EA, O'Higgins R, Mellor DJ, et al. Prevalence and risk factors for feline obesity in a first opinion practice in Glasgow, Scotland. J Feline Med Surg 2010;12(10):746–53.

8. Cave NJ, Allan FJ, Schokkenbroek SL, et al. A cross-sectional study to compare changes in the prevalence and risk factors for feline obesity between 1993 and 2007 in New Zealand. Prev Vet Med 2012;107(1–2):121–33.

9. Michel KE, Anderson W, Cupp C, et al. Correlation of a feline muscle mass score with body composition determined by dual-energy X-ray absorptiometry. Br J Nutr 2011;106(S1):S57–9.

10. German AJ, Holden SL, Bissot T, et al. Use of starting condition score to estimate changes in body weight and composition during weight loss in obese dogs. Res Vet Sci 2009;87:249–54.

11. Laflamme D. Development and validation of a body condition score system for dogs. A clinical tool. Canine Pract 1997;22:10–5.

12. Laflamme D. Development and validation of a body condition score system for cats. A clinical tool. Feline Pract 1997;25:13–8.

13. Courcier EA, Mellor DJ, Pendlebury E, et al. An investigation into the epidemiology of feline obesity in Great Britain: results of a cross-sectional study of 47 companion animal practises. Vet Rec 2012;171(22):560.

14. Mao J, Xia Z, Chen J, et al. Prevalence and risk factors for canine obesity surveyed in veterinary practices in Beijing, China. Prev Vet Med 2013;112(3–4): 438–42.

15. Morrison R, Penpraze V, Beber A, et al. Associations between obesity and physical activity in dogs: a preliminary investigation. J Small Anim Pract 2013;54: 570–4.

16. Rohlf VI, Toukhsati S, Coleman GJ, et al. Dog obesity: can dog caregivers' (owners') feeding and exercise intentions and behaviors be predicted from attitudes? J Appl Anim Welf Sci 2010;13(3):213–36.

17. White GA, Hobson-West P, Cobb K, et al. Canine obesity: is there a difference between veterinarian and owner perception? J Small Anim Pract 2011;52(12): 622–6.

18. Bland IM, Guthrie-Jones A, Taylor RD, et al. Dog obesity: owner attitudes and behavior. Prev Vet Med 2009;92(4):333–40.

19. Corbee RJ. Obesity in show dogs. J Anim Physiol Anim Nutr 2013;97(5):904–10.

20. Murphy M, Lusby AL, Bartges JW, et al. Size of food bowl and scoop affects amount of food owners feed their dogs. J Anim Physiol Anim Nutr 2012;96(2):237–41.

21. German AJ, Holden SL, Mason SL, et al. Imprecision when using measuring cups to weigh out extruded dry kibbled food. J Anim Physiol Anim Nutr 2011; 95(3):368–73.

22. Wang Y, Beydoun MA, Liang L, et al. Will all Americans become overweight or obese? Estimating the progression and cost of the US obesity epidemic. Obesity (Silver Spring) 2008;16:2323–30.

23. Soler GS, Ramos NG, Martinez-Lopez I, et al. Study of drug dose calculation for morbidly obese patients. Farm Hosp 2009;33(6):330–4.

24. Zoran DL. Obesity in dogs and cats: a metabolic and endocrine disorder. Vet Clin North Am Small Anim Pract 2010;40:221–39.

25. Kil DY, Swanson KS. Endocrinology of obesity. Vet Clin North Am Small Anim Pract 2010;40:205–19.

26. Jeusette IC, Lhoest ET, Istasse LP, et al. Influence of obesity on plasma lipid and lipoprotein concentrations in dogs. Am J Vet Res 2005;66(1):81–6.

27. Haring T, Haase B, Zini E, et al. Overweight and impaired insulin sensitivity present in growing cats. J Anim Physiol Anim Nutr 2013;97:813–9.

28. Zoran DL, Rand JS. The role of diet in prevention and management of feline diabetes. Vet Clin North Am Small Anim Pract 2013;43:233–43.

29. Marshall WG, Hazewinkel HA, Mullen D, et al. The effect of weight loss on lameness in obese dogs with osteoarthritis. Vet Res Commun 2010;34:241–53.

30. Clutton RE. The medical implications of canine obesity and their relevance to anaesthesia. Br Vet J 1988;144:21–8.

31. Van Goethem BE, Rosenweldt KW, Kirpensteijn J. Monopolar versus bipolar electrocoagulation in canine laparoscopic ovariectomy: a nonrandomized prospective, clinical trial. Vet Surg 2003;32:464–70.

32. Kealy R, Lawler D, Ballam J, et al. Effects of diet restriction on life span and age-related changes in dogs. J Am Vet Med Assoc 2002;220:1315–20.

33. German AJ, Holden SL, Wiseman-Orr ML, et al. Quality of life is reduced in obese dogs but improves after successful weight loss. Vet J 2012;192(3): 428–34.

34. Van de Velde H, Janssens GP, Rochus K, et al. Proliferation capacity of T-lymphocytes is affected transiently after a long-term weight gain in Beagle dogs. Vet Immunol Immunopathol 2013;152(3–4):237–44.

35. Williams GD, Newberne PM. Decreased resistance to Salmonella infection in obese dogs. Fed Proc 1971;30:572.

36. Nelson RW, Himsel CA, Feldman EC, et al. Glucose tolerance and insulin response in normal weight and obese cats. Am J Vet Res 1990;51:1357–62.

37. Klinkenberg H, Sallander MH, Hedhammar M. Feeding, exercise, and weight identified as risk factors in canine diabetes mellitus. J Nutr 2006;136(7): 1985S–7S.

38. Scarlett JM, Donoghue S. Associations between body condition and disease in cats. J Am Vet Med Assoc 1998;212:1725–31.

39. Gayet C, Bailhache E, Dumon H, et al. Insulin resistance and changes in plasma concentration of TNFalpha, IGF1, and NEFA in dogs during weight gain and obesity. J Anim Physiol Anim Nutr (Berl) 2004;88(3–4):157–65.

40. Hoenig M, Wilkins C, Holson JC, et al. Effects of obesity on lipid profiles in neutered male and female cats. Am J Vet Res 2003;64(3):299–303.

41. Pena C, Suarez L, Bautista I, et al. Relationship between analytic values and canine obesity. J Anim Physiol Anim Nutr (Berl) 2008;92:324–5.

42. Chikamune T, Katamoto H, Ohashi F, et al. Serum lipid and lipoprotein concentrations in obese dogs. J Vet Med Sci 1995;57(4):595–8.

43. Hess RS, Kass PH, Shofer FS, et al. Evaluation of risk factors for fatal acute pancreatitis in dogs. J Am Vet Med Assoc 1999;214:46–51.

44. Smith GK, Mayhew PD, Kapatkin AS, et al. Evaluation of risk factors for degenerative joint disease associated with hip dysplasia in German Shepherd dogs, golden retrievers, Labrador retrievers, and rottweilers. J Am Vet Med Assoc 2001;219:1719–24.

45. van Hagen MA, Ducro BJ, van den Broek J, et al. Incidence, risk factors, and hereditability estimates of hind limb lameness caused by hip dysplasia in a birth cohort of boxers. Am J Vet Res 2005;66:307–12.

46. Impellizeri JA, Tetrick MA, Muir P. Effect of weight reduction on clinical signs of lameness in dogs with hip osteoarthritis. J Am Vet Med Assoc 2000;216: 1089–91.

47. Kealy RD, Lawler DF, Ballam JM, et al. Evaluation of the effect of limited food consumption on radiographic evidence of osteoarthritis in dogs. J Am Vet Med Assoc 2000;217:1678–80.

48. Brown DC, Cozemius MG, Shofer FS. Body weight as a predisposing factor for humeral condylar fractures, cranial cruciate rupture and intervertebral disc disease in cocker spaniels. Vet Comp Orthop Traumatol 1996;9:75–8.

49. Adams P, Bolus R, Middleton S, et al. Influence of signalment on developing cranial cruciate rupture in dogs in the UK. J Small Anim Pract 2011;52(7):347–52.

50. Packer RM, Hendricks A, Volk HA, et al. How long and low can you go? Effect of conformation on the risk of thoracolumbar intervertebral disc extrusion in domestic dogs. PLoS One 2013;8(7):e69650.

51. Litster AL, Buchanan JW. Radiographic and echocardiographic measurement of the heart of obese cats. Vet Radiol Ultrasound 2000;41:320–5.

52. Pelosi A, Rosenstein D, Abood SK, et al. Cardiac effect of short-term experimental weight gain and loss in dogs. Vet Rec 2013;172(6):153.

53. Kuruvilla A, Frankel TL. Heart rate of pet dogs: effects of overweight and exercise. Asia Pac J Clin Nutr 2003;12(S):51.

54. White RA, Williams JM. Tracheal collapse in the dog—is there really a role for surgery? A survey of 100 cases. J Small Anim Pract 1994;35:191–6.

55. Bach JF, Rozanski EA, Bedenice D, et al. Association of expiratory airway dysfunction with marked obesity in healthy adult dogs. Am J Vet Res 2007; 68(6):670–5.

56. Bruchim Y, Klement E, Saragusty J, et al. Heat stroke in dogs: a retrospective study of 54 cases (1999-2004) and analysis of risk factors for death. J Vet Intern Med 2006;20:38–46.

57. Alenza DP, Rutteman GR, Pena L, et al. Relation between habitual diet and canine mammary tumors in a case-control study. J Vet Intern Med 1998;12: 132–9.

58. Glickman LT, Schofer FS, McKee LJ, et al. Epidemiologic study of insecticide exposure, obesity, risk of bladder cancer in household dogs. J Toxicol Environ Health 1989;28:407–14.

59. Tvarijonaviciute A, Ceron JJ, Holden SL, et al. Effect of weight loss in obese dogs on indicators of renal function or disease. J Vet Intern Med 2013;27(1): 31–8.

60. Henegar JR, Bigler SA, Henegar LK, et al. Functional and structural changes in the kidney in the early stages of obesity. J Am Soc Nephrol 2001;12:1211–7.

61. Finco DR, Brown SA, Cooper TA. Effects of obesity on glomerular filtration rate (GFR) in dogs. Compend Contin Educ Pract Vet 2001;23(S):78.

62. Gu JW, Wang J, Stockton A, et al. Cytokine gene expression profiles in kidney medulla and cortex of obese hypertensive dogs. Kidney Int 2004;66:713–21.

63. Lekcharoensuk C, Lulich JP, Osborne CA, et al. Patient and environmental factors associated with calcium oxalate urolithiasis in dogs. J Am Vet Med Assoc 2000;217:515–9.

64. Baldwin K, Bartges J, Buffington T, et al. AAHA nutritional assessment guidelines for dogs and cats. J Am Anim Hosp Assoc 2010;46(4):285–96.

65. Freeman L, Becvarova I, Cave N, et al. WSAVA nutritional assessment guidelines. Compend Contin Educ Vet 2011;33(8):E1–9.

66. Hoenig M, Ferguson DC. Effects of neutering on hormonal concentrations and energy requirements in male and female cats. Am J Vet Res 2002;63(5):634–9.

67. Linder DE, Freeman LM. Evaluation of calorie density and feeding directions for commercially available diets designed for weight loss in cats and dogs. J Am Vet Med Assoc 2010;236(1):74–7.

68. Churchill J. Increase the success of weight loss programs by creating an environment for change. Compend Contin Educ Vet 2010;32(12):E1.

69. Wei A, Fascetti AJ, Villaverde C, et al. Effect of water content in a canned food on voluntary food intake and body weight in cats. Am J Vet Res 2011;72(7): 918–23.

70. Jewell DE, Toll PW, Novotny BJ. Satiety reduces adiposity in dogs. Vet Ther 2000;1(1):17–23.
71. Weber M, Bissot T, Servet E, et al. A high-protein, high-fiber diet designed for weight loss improves satiety in dogs. J Vet Intern Med 2007;21(6):1203–8.
72. Butterwick RF, Hawthorne AJ. Advances in dietary management of obesity in dogs and cats. J Nutr 1998;128(12S):2771S–5S.
73. Yamka RM, Frantz NZ, Friesen KG. Effects of three canine weight loss foods on body composition and obesity markers. Intern J Appl Res Vet Med 2007;5(3): 125–32.
74. Laflamme DP, Hannah SS. Increased dietary protein promotes fat loss and reduces loss of lean body mass during weight loss in cats. Intern J Appl Res Vet Med 2005;3(2):62–8.
75. Backus RC, Cave NJ, Keisler DH. Gonadectomy and high dietary fat but not high dietary carbohydrate induce gains in body weight and fat of domestic cats. Br J Nutr 2007;98(3):641–50.
76. Linder DE, Freeman LM, Morris P, et al. Theoretical evaluation of risk for nutritional deficiency with caloric restriction in dogs. Vet Q 2012;32(3–4):123–9.
77. Linder DE, Freeman LM, Holden SL, et al. Status of selected nutrients in obese dogs undergoing caloric restriction. BMC Vet Res 2013;9:219.
78. Roudebush P, Schoenherr W, Delaney S. An evidence-based review of the use of nutraceuticals and dietary supplementation for the management of obese and overweight pets. J Am Vet Med Assoc 2008;232:1646–55.
79. Bland IM, Guthrie-Jones A, Taylor RD, et al. Dog obesity: veterinary practices' and owners' opinions on cause and management. Prev Vet Med 2010; 94(3–4):310–5.
80. Laflamme DP, Kuhlman G, Lawler DF. Evaluation of weight loss protocols for dogs. J Am Anim Hosp Assoc 1997;33:253–9.
81. Burkholder WJ, Bauer JE. Foods and techniques for managing obesity in companion animals. J Am Vet Med Assoc 1998;212:658–62.
82. Blanchard G, Nguyen P, Gayet C, et al. Rapid weight loss with a high-protein low energy diet allows the recovery of ideal body composition and insulin sensitivity in obese dogs. J Nutr 2004;134:2148S–50S.
83. German AJ, Holden SL, Bissot T, et al. Dietary energy restriction and successful weight loss in obese client-owned dogs. J Vet Intern Med 2007;21:1174–80.
84. Villaverde C, Ramsey J, Green A, et al. Energy restriction results in a mass-adjusted decrease in energy expenditure in cats that is maintained after weight regain. J Nutr 2008;138:856–60.
85. Nagaoka D, Mitsuhashi Y, Angell R, et al. Re-induction of obese body weight occurs more rapidly and at lower caloric intake in beagles. J Anim Physiol Anim Nutr (Berl) 2010;94(3):287–92.
86. Wakshlag JJ, Struble AM, Warren BS, et al. Evaluation of dietary energy intake and physical activity in dogs undergoing a controlled weight-loss program. J Am Vet Med Assoc 2012;240(4):413–9.
87. Chauvet A, Laclair J, Elliot DA, et al. Incorporation of exercise, using an underwater treadmill, and active client education into a weight management program for obese dogs. Can Vet J 2011;52:491–6.
88. Mlacnik E, Bockstahler BA, Müller M, et al. Effects of caloric restriction and a moderate or intense physiotherapy program for treatment of lameness in overweight dogs with osteoarthritis. J Am Vet Med Assoc 2006;229(11):1756–60.
89. Ellis S, Rodan I, Carney H, et al. AAFP and ISFM feline environmental needs guidelines. J Feline Med Surg 2013;15(3):219–30.

90. Phillips K, Wood F, Kinnerley P. Tackling obesity: the challenge of obesity management for practice nurses in primary care. Fam Pract 2014;31(1):51–9.

91. Ogden CL, Carroll MD, Kit BK, et al. Prevalence of obesity in the United States, 2009–2010. NCHS Data Brief 2012;(82):1–8.

92. Herzog HA. Some we love, some we hate, some we eat: why it's so hard to think straight about animals. New York: Harper Collins Publishers; 2010.

93. Budge RC, Spicer J, Jones B, et al. Health correlates of compatibility and attachment in human-companion animal relationships. Soc Anim 1998;6:219–34.

94. Melson GF, Peet S, Sparks C. Children's attachment to their pets: links to socio-emotional development. Child Env Quart 1992;8:55–65.

95. Kurdek LA. Pet dogs as attachment figures for adult owners. J Fam Psychol 2009;23:439–46.

96. Stanley IH, Conwell Y, Bowen C, et al. Pet ownership may attenuate loneliness among older adult primary care patients who live alone. Aging Ment Health 2014;18(3):394–9.

97. Barker SB, Dawson KS. The effects of animal-assisted therapy on anxiety ratings of hospitalized psychiatric patients. Psychiatr Serv 1998;49:797–801.

98. Kushner RF, Blatner DJ, Jewell DE, et al. The PPET Study: people and pets exercising together. Obesity (Silver Spring) 2006;14(10):1762–70.

99. Stephens MB, Wilson CC, Goodie JL, et al. Health perceptions and levels of attachment: owners and pets exercising together. J Am Board Fam Med 2012;25(6):923–6.

Index

Note: Page numbers of article titles are in **boldface** type.

Vet Clin Small Anim 44 (2014) 807–816
http://dx.doi.org/10.1016/S0195-5616(14)00076-X
0195-5616/14/$ – see front matter © 2014 Elsevier Inc. All rights reserved.

Printed and bound by CPI Group (UK) Ltd, Croydon, CR0 4YY

03/10/2024

01040497-0015